MY ONLINE ANGEL

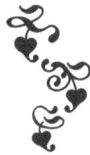

Jonathan Greeson

MILVERSTEAD PUBLISHING

Philadelphia

ISBN-13: 978-0-9842847-9-5

ISBN-10: 0-9842847-9-6

Cover and interior design
by Joel Friedlander and Zoe Lonergan
www.TheBookDesigner.com

Milverstead Publishing LLC
31 Rampart Drive
Wayne, PA 19087
(888)667-3981

Visit us on the web!

www.milversteadpublishing.com

Foreword

THE FOLLOWING STORY IS BASED on a true event that I experienced in my life. However, the names have been changed to protect the identities of the characters involved. I share this story because I believe we can all use it to look at our own personal relationships. Too often in life we are led by fear of rejection in our pursuit of love, which leads us to unhappy relationships because we settle. However, we still engage in the pursuit of love and happiness because in the bottom of our hearts we know that it is still out there. This story happened to me in a time where I was almost ready to stop that pursuit, but an angel came into my life to remind me that I was good enough to keep waiting for that illusive "perfect" woman we all hope to find. I hope that our story reminds you to be relentless in your pursuit as well.

I also hope that this story helps break down a barrier for people with disabilities. Being disabled, I know from first-hand experience that dating is the hardest obstacle we face in life. It sounds silly with all the obstacles we face, but building a ramp or writing a new law for equal rights is easy. Try getting a young person to look past your wheelchair and see you as a person worth spending the rest of their life with, now that is a true challenge. There are no laws to help you get a person to fall in love with you. You have to be able to ease their own fears while handling your own demons of lack of self-confidence. There was a time when I didn't believe a person would ever be able to see past my disability enough for a relationship, but now I know better. I hope this story helps others realize their own potential in the dating world and all other aspects of life.

Chapter 1

❧

☙

ANSWERED PRAYER

I HAVE LIVED A GOOD LIFE. I have a great family and great friends who support everything I do. They are always there when I pursue my goals, which I attain because of their support. What makes it special is that for me to do anything, I have to have help from those closest to me. I have a genetic condition called Spinal Muscular Atrophy, which is a type of Muscular Dystrophy that causes me to be confined to a wheelchair. I've never been one to dwell on that or use my condition as an excuse, so I pursued the same goals as all of my other able-bodied friends as we grew up. This included graduating from high school and earning a bachelor's degree from a major university. I also developed a love for sports at a very young age, which led me to an internship in professional hockey and helped me start a hockey program for people who use wheelchairs. Of course, achieving all of these goals has been difficult, but they are not impossible, as some people in my situation would believe.

With all of the good things that are in my life, there has always been something missing. We all want someone to share our lives with. It's just natural. When you have a good day at work or school, you want to come home and share that moment with your significant other. Some relationships don't work out that way, but I have always believed in romance and true love. There have been many women I have been interested in over the years, and it always seems to end up the same way. They think of me as a great friend, but never any more than that.

I think that happens a lot when there is a disability involved. First, from my side, I cannot just lean in and kiss a girl I'm interested in because most of the time I am sitting at butt level. Most girls don't really like guys to literally "kiss their ass." Think about a person sitting down beside you while you are standing, and you can see my point. Of course, we all know a girl never makes the first move. I think that would be a dream come true for any guy! So, when I'm interested in a girl, I'm kind of screwed (and not in the good way) because I really cannot take the initiative. I do understand that there are other circumstances that make dating a person with a disability a little more complicated and, yes, almost scary. I would have the same concerns if I were in their position. Human nature makes us afraid of the unknown. However, our society prevents us from asking questions because it isn't "politically correct."

It's funny to me how guys are often referred to as "pigs" or "disgusting" when they are sexually attracted to a woman, but from what I have learned in my own life experiences, women are the exact same way. Although they won't admit it, they want to get laid as much as a man does. They just may keep these feelings to themselves. I have known girls who really liked me and would even consider dating me, but as they thought about the future, the sex question would come into their mind. However, instead of talking about it and figuring things out, it was time for us to be just friends.

So, Ladies, let me take a moment to enlighten you. I'm not sure about all disabilities, but most of us have full function "down there" and there are medications to help those who don't. We just have to be a little more creative and careful with how we have sex. Communication is the key to any relationship, so this is just another topic for you to talk about with your partner. Able-bodied people talk about their likes/dislikes in the bedroom, so why should it be any different for a person with a disability? Of course, sex may not be an option for some of us, but should you really throw away a chance at happiness because of that? I understand the desire to have a family, but there are alternatives, such as adoption. As we grow older, shouldn't the lifelong companionship be worth more than a little fun in the bedroom?

There are actually a couple of advantages to being with a guy with a disability. The first is we know that you are coming out of your comfort zone to be with us, so we will appreciate you more than other guys. Also, you are in complete control in the bedroom and I've heard that's a welcome change for most women. Of course, I'm not promoting just going out and hooking up with a guy in a wheelchair for the fun of it. If he is like me, he has enough to worry about and doesn't want to add an STD to that list, so you wouldn't have a chance until we were in love. I'm telling you this so you won't just pass up a chance at true happiness because you are afraid of the unknown. Yes, it can be a little difficult to start your life with someone you already have to take care of, but what if you loved an able-bodied guy who suddenly had an accident and was paralyzed; would you love him any less? Would you leave that guy just because your "perfect" little home was altered? If so, then you weren't really in love, anyway. Well, you may have been in love with the idea of love and marriage, but you were not in love with that specific person if you can just replace him with another guy who can walk.

Some people want to get married and that's it, but I want to find that one person with whom I am truly meant to be. I want that person who will be even more beautiful to me 50 years from now than she is today, someone to whom I can leave a single rose and she would gush like I gave her the world instead of asking where the other 11 are. Someone who doesn't care how much was spent on a date as long as we are spending time together. It is rare to find someone like that, but I have always believed they do exist. All the love stories and movies have to be based on something.

There was a time recently when I stopped believing that one day

I could find this happiness. It wasn't that I thought there was something wrong with me, but I started to believe that there was no way a woman would ever be able to get over the fact that I am in a wheelchair. I was to the point that I would just wait until I was middle-aged when women have stopped looking for the guy who was fun to go to clubs with and show off to their friends and started looking for that life-long friend to share their life with. It's funny how when you think you have all the time in the world to wait, God sends a message to remind you that your time on this Earth is limited.

I don't believe His message to me was to start looking for a date, but I do believe that now I should be loving every moment of my life and not waiting for things to come to me.

I caught the flu, which doesn't sound like much, but when you have a disability, it can be deadly. My flu resulted in pneumonia, and before I knew what happened, I was in the emergency room having an emergency tracheotomy. The doctors tried to intubate me, but they couldn't get my mouth opened enough. They even knocked out my two front teeth. I remember that moment, but then I passed out and was in a coma for 2 weeks. I will never tell all of the dreams I had during that time, but I do know it was the scariest time of my life. I finally awoke to an empty room as my parents were unable to be in the room with me at the time. I was on a ventilator and feeding tube and could not talk. I have never felt so lost in my life, but that was just the beginning. I spent 44 days in the intensive care unit. Luckily, my doctor wrote a prescription allowing my parents to stay in the room with me. The nurses were good, but I was a special situation, and my family knew my needs better than anyone, especially being I couldn't talk. It took me about three months to get all the tubes out of me, and eventually I started getting all my strength back. It's amazing how you have to have a near-death experience like that to realize life is too short. We never know when we're going to be taken from this world.

I had a few more experiences talking to girls and ending up just being friends as usual after my illness. It was the same old story; the girl isn't as honest with me as she should be because she doesn't want to hurt me, so I end up getting hurt. I always remain friends with them, which sounds crazy, but they just didn't know any better. Plus, I think it's a good quality in a friend if they try everything to keep you from getting hurt whether it be physical or emotional pain. After my hospital stay, however, I decided that I was tired of playing that "game." I didn't want to waste a prayer on asking God to send me a girlfriend because I think He has more important things to do, but I did ask for just one person to be honest with me and I would take care of the rest. I just wanted to know that it was possible for me to be loved by someone in that way. It was exactly 10 days later that my prayer was answered.

Chapter 2

❧

MOLLY

I'M A MEMBER OF THE online social networking sites. They are a great way to keep up with old friends, but sometimes you can meet new people, too. However, sometimes strangers who pop up as friend requests are just wanting you to go to another site and see their nude photos, so you have to be careful.

This is how Molly came into my life. I checked my page one morning and had a friend request from a cute girl named Molly. Of course, I believed it was just a scam at first, so I looked at her page to see what crazy excuse she had come up with to try and get me to look at her "personal" photos. To my surprise, there were only photos of her with friends and family. I was really confused because I had no clue who Molly was; I was worried I might have forgotten her because of my illness. I had already realized that some things slipped from my mind during my coma.

I decided to send her a message mainly to see how she knew me, but also because I thought she was adorable and wanted to get to know her if we hadn't met. She had the most beautiful blue eyes that I could stare at all day. I knew that if she was real, I had to meet her. What did I have to lose? She was online, so it wasn't like I would see her everyday if something didn't work out. For the first time in my life, I wasn't afraid of being rejected, but I was still skeptical of whether or not she was real.

I sent her a message and she replied the next day that we didn't know each other. Her friend, Maggie, had talked her into social networking to meet new people as she didn't like to go to clubs. I was already excited because I finally found a girl in her twenties whose social life didn't revolve around loud music and alcohol. I don't have anything against that type of activity, but it's not my favorite way to meet people. Again, I'm looking for that best friend to share my life with, not just a one-night stand. Honesty is important to me, and while it's rare online, it's just as rare in clubs. Not to mention online is not as loud or uncomfortable, and it's less expensive than going out to a club.

We started casually sending messages and just finding out about each other. It was the typical small talk as you would have with any person of the opposite sex. We all send out those "feeler" questions to help us find out whether or not they have a boy-friend and whether or not they are interested in you. It's the same way online, but you can't read the reactions of the person. You can't see the smile or hear the laugh at your joke, nor can you see the body actions to help you know if the person is interested. For example, we all know that when a girl crosses her arms to talk to you, she's "closing herself up" and you don't have a chance. I have also learned that the other universal signal is if a girl casually calls you "bud." If a girl ever says, "Hey bud," to you, there is absolutely no way you will ever date her, so just quit trying.

I'll never understand why it is easier to talk to someone online because you cannot see the signs - maybe because we don't want that person to see our reaction when we get rejected? It's hard to believe we will never take chances because we are worried about being embarrassed. Who really cares if a guy approaches a goddess and she rejects him? If anything, I'm proud of him! He had the guts to do something nobody else would do. There is actually a really good chance that she's single and may give you a shot. It's not like you have to get married, anyway.

That was my theory with Molly. She was my goddess, and I was going to approach her the best way I could, which was online. She was a dental hygienist, so I considered knocking out my teeth again and going to her office to have them fixed, but I decided it would be safer to just email her. It was amazing! We started with the casual conversation but were able to really open up with each other rather quickly. She soon became a major part of my day as I had an email waiting for me in the morning. She left for work earlier than I did, and she was one of those strange people who actually enjoy mornings. I started to refer to her as my "morning coffee" because I got to where I couldn't start my day without her. I would then make sure to have an email waiting for her when she got home from work and then we would exchange a couple of emails in the evening before going to sleep. There was a time when I had 1500 saved emails from Molly.

So everything was going great. I had finally found a girl I wasn't afraid of and with whom I could be honest. I also started to trust her. I'll be the first to admit that I do have serious trust issues with women because I have had too many experiences with women just being nice to me so I wouldn't get hurt. I finally started to get over that with her because our "relationship" wasn't just me doing all the work, she was always there as the first person I heard from in the morning and the last at night. A girl wouldn't put that time in if she was just being nice.

I even discovered that Molly and I had the same type of sense of humor, which I believe was part of the reason we connected so quickly. I can be sarcastic, and I like to pick and play with people. Some people can handle that and some get offended way too easily. It was great because Molly even started to play little practical jokes on me.

One night we got on the subject of what we were the most comfortable sleeping in. I always sleep in some pajama pants and a t-shirt, so my comments on the subject weren't very exciting.

Molly had a little more fun with me, though. First, being the tease that she was, she said she was most comfortable sleeping in the nude. Then she added that she liked to sleep in silk lingerie just because it made her feel more like a woman and a little sexy. I decided to have a little fun with that and said that I would love to see that and told her to send me a picture. Of course, I knew she wouldn't do it, but it was still fun to ask. Maggie had already told her the rule of online dating where you never do anything where people have proof of your actions. I never forgave Maggie for that. She ruined all my fun! Anyway, the next day I had an email from Molly and the subject said "What is your favorite color?-PRIVATE." The email was also a large file, which meant that it had to be pictures. I was shocked that she actually did it! I wasn't even sure if I should open it, it just felt wrong. I eventually did open it when I was alone, which was great because I laughed so hard! Each picture file had a color…green, pink, red, black, etc. I opened the green one first because it was the first picture. To my surprise there was this really pretty piece of green silk lingerie on the hanger of her bedroom door. Of course, she wasn't in the picture! I knew there was no way she would actually send me a dirty photo. She was such a tease, but that was probably one of the best jokes ever done to me. I still laugh when I think about it.

Of course, I was still a little skeptical that my online dream girl could be a man, someone in prison, a crazy woman wanting to molest a person with a disability, or a scam trying to get access to my bank account. Yes, I definitely have trust issues. I knew it wasn't a scam after about 2 weeks because she never asked for anything. A con artist will not invest that much time in a person. The only way to solve the other mysteries about Molly was to meet her. It would have to be a public place because I wasn't letting her know where I lived just in case she was that crazy woman with a disability fetish. I decided to ask her to meet me somewhere, which she wanted to do, but she didn't want to officially meet yet. She was, however, open and honest as to why we couldn't meet at that time.

༄

Chapter 3

BAGGAGE

*I*T SEEMS LIKE EVERY TIME I meet a sweet girl, my timing is always wrong. Of course, sometimes it is a girl's way of rejecting you, but sometimes you really can just meet at the wrong time. The same problem happened yet again with Molly. She was single, but she was recently out of a long-term relationship and wasn't completely over the guy yet.

James was the first guy that she had ever been with; they started dating in high school. They stayed together through college and continued their relationship into their respective careers. They were still together but were growing apart. It happens to everyone. We all change as we get older. Molly was still with him mainly because it was comfortable and she was used to having him in her life.

Although he was in her life, he wasn't really there for her. Molly's mother became sick with cancer and when she needed that shoulder to cry on, he was never available. When he was available, they just argued because he couldn't understand what she was going through. They finally decided to end their relationship after six years, and Molly sank into a deep depression and wouldn't do anything. That was when Maggie talked her into signing up for a social networking site and ordered her to add some friends so she could meet new people.

Molly would later admit to me that she added me because my page is mostly related to promoting my wheelchair hockey team, so she thought I would be safe. She was terrified of meeting a person online even though it was how Maggie met her current boyfriend. Honestly, I was afraid of meeting Molly as well. Again, I still didn't know if she was a man, a convict, or a crazy person with a wheelchair fetish. However, I was able to hide my concerns by being a nice guy and giving her time to get over the last guy as well as both of us get over our fears.

That plan, however, backfired on me because James came back in her life. He gave her the same old story of wanting to try again and how he couldn't live without her. Of course, my translation for that story is "I went looking around for other girls and I couldn't get laid, so I need to come back to you." Usually, when something like this happens, girls try to hide it from me, but Molly was up front and honest with me. She explained how she was really glad we found each other online, but she felt like she owed it to him because of their past. I really admired the fact that she didn't try to hide it, so I told her I understood and had no problem with it. She needed to go and see if there was anything left between them before she could really move on, but I also reminded her that her first love didn't have to be her last. I wasn't saying that I was "the one" for her, but she should never settle just because James was the only guy she has ever loved.

Some guys would have moved on to the next girl, but I really enjoyed talking to her and I knew I had her interested in seeing who else was out there. I would later tell her that I knew I had her at the metaphorical fence, but it was her decision whether or not to cross over and see if the grass was really greener on the other side. Until she made that decision, I at least had someone new to talk to. The other advantage of keeping her in my life was the confidence she gave me. While I would never cheat on a woman, it does give you confidence to have another person in your "back pocket" while you are playing the dating game. We all have a fear of being alone, which can be the root of low self-esteem. Therefore, we hold in our feelings of attraction to the opposite sex, so they will at least continue to talk to us. However, when you know that there is another person in your back pocket available to talk to, you can be more confident and take more chances. The same theory can be true in all parts of life. In hockey for example, you have confidence in your goaltender that he will be there to keep the other team from scoring, so you will force the puck up the ice and try to score. If the goaltender wasn't there, would you still try to score or would you try to defend? Dating is the same; would you rather defend your confidence and be shy or would rather put it all on the line? Everyone knows you will never score a goal if you don't ever take a shot. I'm not the only person who does it, either. The next time you talk to a girl, notice her confidence around you. If she isn't shy at all, you can be about 90% sure she isn't single.

Although I'm not really proud of it, I used the same theory with Molly. What else could I do? I had to wait and see what happened with the other guy, but I wasn't getting any younger and had to live my life. I did notice a huge boost to my confidence with girls. I have always set the bar high with everything I have done, and my expectations aren't any different with girls. I believe that a woman can be smart, sweet, and beautiful, and I will not settle for any less. One of those characteristics alone is not enough, nor are they the only three I look for, but they get my attention. Of course, I have to be honest and admit physical attractiveness is the first characteristic I notice, as does everyone else. There is no way to look at a person across the room and know what types of values they have. You can look at their clothes and other accessories to get an idea, but what makes you approach them is part of their physical appearance. Whether it be an attractive body, beautiful eyes, or an amazing smile, it's still a trigger from their physical beauty. We all have different preferences and everyone is beautiful in their own way, but it is the first thing we notice. I do not believe that makes me shallow because every person does it. I am just willing to admit it. This is true in other parts of life as well. Have you ever gone to a job interview with ragged clothes and actually been offered the job? No, the job interviewer makes a judgment on your physical appearance, although they aren't supposed to.

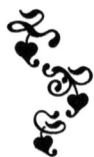

Chapter 4

❧

QUESTIONS

*T*HE TRUTH IS, HOWEVER, THAT I always knew that I wouldn't really pursue any other relationships until I found out what would happen with Molly. My friends almost felt sorry for me because they thought she was leading me on and we would never meet. I realize it does sound crazy to wait around for a girl you have never physically seen, but I had my reasons. The biggest reason was that she never tried to hide things from me. She also had the same concerns that other girls had regarding how far our relationship could go. However, instead of running away, she asked me straight up when she had a question. I knew that she had never even met a person with a disability, so I told her if she ever had any questions, not to hesitate to ask me. I would let her know if it was offensive. Of course, after a lifetime of having strangers check me out from head to toe and help me with all my daily needs such as bathing and using the bathroom, it takes a lot to offend me. One of her biggest fears was that she would hurt me during sex, which was hilarious to me because I was just excited to have a girl thinking about sleeping with me! After I got my composure, I explained to her that I couldn't answer that because I honestly didn't know what would happen, but I was more than willing to try. She was shocked to find out how inexperienced I was in the physical aspects of a relationship, but I've never been one to see women as a toy to play with. My mom and 2 older sisters raised me to respect women and not pursue them as a sport. I want to be in love and be sure she loves me back before I do anything like that. I really am one of those old-fashioned guys who prefer to wait until marriage, but I'm also realistic in that with today's society, sex is a major part of a relationship and I believe a girl has the right to be sure I can keep her happy before she goes into a marriage. Dating is like a job interview and there is nothing wrong with her wanting to be sure you can do all parts of the job before she "hires" you.

While I sound noble waiting for the right person, major reasons I don't sleep around are purely related to my disability. I cannot drive a car, so it really doesn't work to well to have your mom drive you to a hotel to meet a woman. I have to put the time in to building a relationship to a point where I can trust the woman to drive me somewhere without the assistance of my friends or family members. The other fear I have is being left in a hotel bed for three days because a strange woman lured me into a room and robbed me once I was out of my chair. Most people don't realize it, but when you have a disability like mine, your life is often put in the hands of others. Therefore, it is vital that you trust them, especially if in a vulnerable position.

Of course, Molly wasn't all about sex. She also asked me questions about my daily living. She wanted to be completely prepared as to what she would need to do during a day to help me. I was amazed that she was thinking that far ahead when we have never even met. However, she also had the same belief in that there was no reason to pursue a relationship if you knew it would never end up in marriage or at least enough of a commitment to live together. We talked about everything from helping me get breakfast in the morning to putting my bipap respiratory machine on before going to bed at night. I really began to admire her for having such a strong desire to help me. I started to believe that I finally found someone so wonderful that she could look past my wheelchair and see the guy she knew she has always wanted.

Unfortunately, during this wonderful time of getting to know each other, the other guy was still trying to see her. At that time, I really had no right to say she couldn't see him. Honestly, I wanted her to see him just to make sure there was nothing there. Maybe it was a self-confidence issue for me, I'm not sure, but I did know that it would be very tough for me to actually compete with another guy to be with her. I didn't think James was better than me, but again, for a woman to date someone with a disability, she has to come out of her comfort zone. Not only was

I competing with a guy who could walk, but I was also dealing with the fact that for 6 years, this guy was all that Molly knew. How could I make her give that up for a chance at me when we may or may not work out? What if we got along great, but she couldn't handle having to take care of me? If that happened, would she take the easy way out and go back to the guy who was comfortable?

I actually talked to Molly about the issues going through my head because I decided if we were going to have any chance at all, she had to be sure there was nothing between her and James. I didn't want her to choose a guy just because he was able to do yard work or change the oil in a car. From what I have seen with my family and their own marriages, some of their main arguments come from their husbands not doing physical labor, so I was paranoid that these issues could keep me from ever finding happiness. I know there are more things to having a "happy home," but I knew that the ability to do chores was one thing that James could give Molly, and I couldn't. I'll never forget what she said to me when I told her about these concerns. She took a moment to gather her thoughts and said, "Jonathan, that's why they have all these landscaping companies and mechanics. There are too many other things that you do to make me happy for me to worry about the very few things you can't do." It was at that time that I really started to fall for Molly. Finally, someone had come into my life who could see the positives through the negative. Too often in our society, people focus on the negative. For example, when someone wins $100 million in the lottery, the first thing someone says is, "Well they have to pay $50 Million in taxes." Think about it, if someone told you that you could give them a dollar in order to win $100 Million, but you have to give half of it back, wouldn't you happily give that dollar? Personally, I believe that would be a joyous occasion, and I would gladly give half of it back. Molly was so refreshing in that she could see the positive in just about everything, which is something I try to do and is a trait I look for in people.

After our conversation, I started to believe I was getting into a real relationship. Of course, then I also got scared. Some may call it a fear of commitment, but I don't think it's that. I believe it's more of fear of the unknown. I am great at the flirting and the one or two dates where you don't really know what the other person is expecting. After that, we would start getting in to the uncomfortable area where the girl didn't know what to do with me, therefore starting the dishonesty. That is the point where all my past "relationships" ended. Again, all I've ever wanted was someone to be honest with me. While I may not be strong physically, I am really strong emotionally. A girl's making a choice and not being interested in me will not kill me; there are bigger tragedies in life. However, people don't know that and they believe they are doing the right thing by trying not to hurt me. You cannot fault a person for that.

Some may say that Molly was being worse than the other girls because she was openly seeing the other guy, but I completely disagree. Yes, they did see each other, but she didn't try to hide it and I also truly believed that nothing was happening on their "dates." James was getting extremely frustrated because she wouldn't go ahead and start dating him again. She was able to buy time by saying he hurt her so bad the last time that it would take her a while to trust him again. I really tried my best not to influence her decision, but you could tell the only reason she was hesitant in taking him back was that she now knew the world had other possibilities. Granted, that was great news for me, but I started to feel bad about stealing her away from him. He didn't know about me, so it almost felt like I was in the middle of an affair. Technically, she was single and I had every right to talk to her, but my conscience was killing me!

Chapter 5

❦

THE WAITING GAME

*M*OLLY SAW JAMES ONLY ON weekends and always during the day such as for a walk at the park. She didn't allow him to visit during the week because she wanted to take her time deciding which guy she wanted. The weekdays were great because we talked all the time, and I knew she didn't see him. However, the weekends were tough because by Sunday evening, all my trust and confidence issues were taking over. Although I believed nothing was happening, I couldn't stand the fact that he got to see her and I couldn't. I knew that if things kept progressing like this, I was just going to get too attached and get hurt. I also started to realize that it wasn't fair to anyone for me to be involved in their situation. I never wanted to be the guy who stole a girl from anyone, so I decided I would back away. It was just the right thing to do for everyone.

On Monday while Molly was at work, I decided to send an email, not with the intention of ending it completely, but letting her know that I wouldn't be in the way. I assured her that if she ever wanted to try something with me, I would be there as long as I was still single.

I heard from her that night, and she was very upset. She said she had a feeling in her gut that something bad was going to happen that day, but she didn't think I would be "breaking up" with her. She then continued to say that she was so glad she was able to get to know me and that I was a blessing in her life. She understood what I was doing but wished I didn't feel it was necessary. I explained that I wasn't breaking up with her, I was just backing away to protect myself, as I knew I was falling for her.

Over the next few days, we still talked and my morning email was always waiting for me. How could I just sit there and let her go? What if she was brought into my life for a reason?

Our little "break-up" lasted all of two days. No matter how hard I tried, I couldn't go without talking to her, and she was always there to respond. I did decide however, that if I was going to dive back into this situation, then we had to meet. I wasn't worried about her being completely over the other guy anymore. However, she still didn't know what she wanted to do. She said she knew that once we met, she wouldn't want to leave me at all. That really scared her because although she was beautiful and we got along great online, she was afraid she wouldn't be good enough for me in reality. I admit I do have high standards, but everyone should have high standards in choosing a mate. Marriage is the single most important decision of your life and shouldn't be taken lightly. I would much rather spend the rest of my life single than to be miserable because I settled.

Although I tried my best to make her comfortable enough to meet, she didn't want to until James was gone. She wanted to end it with him, but there was a timing issue. Molly didn't have many close friends, and one of them had been begging her to visit her for a weekend. Of course, she wanted Molly to bring James to hang out with her fiancé, his best friend throughout high school. I've often heard about "couple friends" that are really only friends with you because you are dating someone they know. Then when you ever break up with that person, those friends are gone. Personally, that's not my idea of a true friend, but a lot of people get stuck in those situations.

I truly believe that some guys even use those situations to keep girlfriends. I believe James was doing this with Molly. He started to realize that he was losing Molly, so he avoided seeing her alone, when it would be the perfect chance for her to end their relationship. By being nice to her in front of people, he was able to have those people support him. He even went so far as to send flowers to work for no reason. It sounds like a sweet thing to do, but they would have had the same effect sent to her house. He sent them to the office, though, so everyone there could tell her how sweet he was and keep the pressure on her not to leave him.

I was very proud of Molly because she didn't fall for these little tricks. Of course, it helped that I told her what he was doing. She asked me how I knew, and I told her because that's what I would do if I were James. I'm a nice guy, but I admit that I can be manipulative and turn situations to make sure they benefit me. It's not a great trait, but dating is like a job interview; you have to do everything you can to be the best option to the interviewer. The other guy's games were allowing him to get "references" because people were able to see how nice he was treating her.

After all of James' tricks failed, he called the friend to see why Molly was being so noncommittal. James asked her if Molly was seeing someone else because every time he talked about going to visit their friends, Molly would change the subject or say she couldn't get away that weekend. While she wanted to see her friends, she knew that I wouldn't like it at all if she went on this little weekend getaway. She talked to her mother and a family friend about it. They decided that she had to tell James about me. As much as she was holding back with James, it was obvious she had strong feelings for me. The family friend told her to go spend a weekend with him with their friends and then spend a weekend with me. Then she would be able to make her decision.

While I liked the idea of finally getting to meet Molly, I wasn't a fan of this plan at all because I felt like a car she was taking out for a test drive. I wasn't going to spend that whole weekend wondering if I made her happier than he did. I was already at a disadvantage because they were going to be with friends who wanted them to be together, so they would help him put the pressure on her. I guessed that perfectly because as soon as she told him about me, the first thing he said was, "Well before you meet him can we go visit our friends?" He also pulled the typical "I deserve it because I didn't treat you like I should have" and the "You can never really appreciate something until you don't have it anymore" spiels as any guy would when he knows a girl is leaving him.

I knew that this trip was his last ditch effort to try and hang on to Molly, and he knew it as well. Molly knew I didn't want her to go, but I gave her my blessing. If that was what it took for me to meet her, then I was fine with her going. I knew we couldn't talk during that time, so I asked her to have Maggie let me know that she made it there safely. After all, it was Maggie's fault we got into this dilemma, and she needed to do some work!

I admit I was a little scared that I would lose Molly after this weekend, but I really think that was more of the self-confidence issues than anything else. I knew in my heart that Molly was coming back and she would be ready to meet. She was a different person now, and while all of her friends may have still been living in the high school past, Molly had grown into a mature woman and was ready to see what the world had to offer.

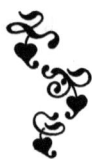

Chapter 6

PHONE CALL

*B*EFORE WE KNEW WHAT HAPPENED, it was time for the weekend trip. It was strange because although I knew she was spending the weekend with James, I was so excited because in less than a week, I was going to meet Molly. It was almost like Christmas! The plan was for them to leave Saturday morning early and be home Sunday evening. Sunday night we were going to have our first phone conversation, and later in the week we were going to meet at a local restaurant for a dessert. We lived about 40 miles from each other, so I suggested a restaurant that was just about halfway between us. Both of us knew we would be nervous, so we decided not to waste money on a whole meal that we wouldn't be able to eat. My weight is also a concern with my disability and missing a meal can make me feel very weak. I would eat before going on the date just to be safe. The last thing

I wanted was to pass out the first time we met.

We had waited on the phone conversation for a couple of reasons. First, I didn't want to talk to her until she decided what was going to happen between her and James. I did want to talk to her before we actually met just to be sure she wasn't a man, but I knew if I heard her voice, she would become too real for me, and then I would be way too attached. I was already falling for her, so I didn't need to do anything to allow me to get hurt any worse if it didn't work out. We always have to keep our guard up.

I also had concerns about the phone conversation because I have a minor speech impediment due to my disability. It's not that I can't talk, I just have a very low voice, and people occasionally have a hard time hearing me. It has never really been a big concern of mine until I started going to job interviews. I majored in finance and wanted to be a financial advisor, but that didn't work out because of lack of experience. I tried to gain experience by applying for a government job, which really shot my confidence with my voice over the phone. The guy interviewed me and everything was going great and then he said there would be a lot of phone calls with vendors and he noticed I didn't have the clearest speaking abilities. At that point I knew I didn't have the job, but the guy went on asking me if I thought I could do the job. Being the smart ass that I am, I looked right at him and said, "Look, I know not to apply to be a truck driver, but there is no doubt in my mind that I can do this job."

I didn't want Molly to be all excited about meeting me and then hear my voice and freak out or something. Granted, I knew that would never happen, but again, I was just being paranoid. Lucky for me, Molly felt the same way about the phone in that we needed to wait until we were ready to meet and really pursue our relationship. We did talk every day, so not having her number was really no big deal to me.

Honestly, I really preferred email because it was another way for us to truly get to know each other. Remember, in order for Molly to be comfortable dating me, I had to get her to see past the wheelchair and get to know me as a person. With a phone and caller ID, people can choose whether or not to listen to you or even answer the phone. Therefore, they are already making a judgment about you before you even have a chance. By using email, you are more likely to be able to lure a person in with your words. When you send a resume in for a job, you include a cover letter that allows you to sell your values to the company. The same concept can be used in an email. Please understand that I don't consider it a way to trick someone into falling for you, but rather a way of helping you get her to look past your disability. In matters of the heart, there are no laws or equality; it's our job to show someone that we can love and it is okay for them to love us back. You cannot do that by leaving a 30- second voicemail. By writing an email, you can take your time, get your thoughts together, and maybe say that one thing that convinces her you are worth it.

The weekend flew by, fortunately, because I had plans that weekend. On Saturday I had hockey practice, which is always an all-day event to get all the equipment in the gym and plan everything. That night I was able to go to a baseball game with one of my best friends and I had family in town to distract me on Sunday. It was amazing how I had no concern at all about Molly's being away with the other guy. My best friend and I spent the baseball game discussing the plans for meeting Molly as he would be driving me to see her. My family didn't know about Molly at that time, so I couldn't really ask my mom or dad to take me on a blind date.

A blind date with someone I felt I already knew.

Chapter 7

❦

MOLLY IS MISSING

FINALLY, IT WAS SUNDAY NIGHT. I went to my bedroom with my phone so I could be alone when I received Molly's call. There was a game on, so as far as anyone in my house was concerned, I was watching that. I waited by the phone until 11:00 and never received a call. Immediately, I started remembering all my past experiences with women, and I became very angry. I was mad at her because I thought she was better than they were, and I was really mad at myself for falling for the same crap again. How could I keep putting myself through this pain, especially when I didn't even know if Molly was real? I don't know why, but for some reason, my heart and my gut were telling me to calm down. I didn't want to listen, but then I remembered that I asked for Molly to come into my life. I shouldn't just brush her off and move on to the next one. Not to mention

I felt a real connection with Molly where I didn't feel like I had anything to prove to her. She liked me for me. I didn't want to just throw that away.

I knew that Molly had to be at work on Monday, so I decided to wait and see if I got my morning email. Maybe the other guy didn't leave on time and they were late getting home? Or maybe they fell back in love and she just couldn't tell me? I had many thoughts going through my head, but I tried to stay positive. I knew she was too good a person to just let me go without any closure. After I didn't get my morning email, I decided to email Maggie to see what was wrong.

She said that she hadn't heard anything from Molly and was truly shocked that Molly hadn't contacted me. She and Molly had talked prior to the trip and she believed Molly was more excited about meeting me than anything else. She only went on the trip so she could meet me with a clear conscience. Once I heard that, all the anger faded away; however, it was replaced by fear. I knew something was wrong, and Maggie said she would make some calls to get us some answers.

And Maggie got them. As they were leaving to come home, Molly was in an accident. Another car ran the stoplight and t-boned them. The car was destroyed, and James was really banged up. His injuries would cause him to stay in the hospital for a very long time. Molly had some cuts, bruises, and a mild concussion, but she would be okay. Of course, her emotions were all screwed up after a near-death experience. Molly's parents told Maggie that they were going to be with Molly and would call her with updates. She would then relay the messages to me.

This was a very trying time for me because a girl I cared for very deeply was hurting and I couldn't be with her. I would have done anything just to hold her, but I knew it would have been bad of me to show up as James was lying there in a hospital bed. I have been in that bed before and I knew that was the last thing he needed. I also started to worry that his injury would cause Molly to see that she didn't want a guy she had to take care of. However, Maggie told me that maybe the accident happened to show Molly she could take care of someone. Like Molly, Maggie was also good at finding a positive in everything. Maggie also took that moment to yell at me and told me to stop feeling sorry for myself. Molly had told her how strong and mature I was, so I needed to act like it. This accident was just a little speed bump in the road that was our relationship.

For about a week Maggie continued to give me updates when Molly's parents would call. She was even able to talk to Molly for a few minutes on the phone. Maggie told Molly how concerned I was, but that I was handling things all right. Molly was really concerned about me because she didn't know what was going to happen and that I wouldn't be there when she finally came home. Of course, Maggie told her she didn't think I was going anywhere.

The next week, Molly's parents came home to get her some extra clothes and take care of things around the house. She decided that she was going to stay up there until James came home. I didn't like that decision at first, but again, I have been in that bed before, too. I was not going to have her come home and we start dating while he was up there alone. It just wasn't right. The accident happened in a different state, so they didn't know the doctors or anything. James needed a familiar face to keep him from going insane. His parents were there, but it's always nice to have some friends as well when in that situation. Of course, those other "friends" who just had to see them went on living their lives as if nothing happened. They did visit for an hour or so during the weekdays, but on the weekends when they could be visiting, they were always traveling and living their lives.

It didn't take long for Maggie to make her way up to visit Molly. The next time Molly's parents went back, Maggie rode with them to surprise Molly. I knew Molly would be so happy to see her, but I was really happy because Maggie was taking a laptop to her! Before they left for the trip, we'd started doing online chats instead of just emails. We would talk nightly for over 2 hours. I hadn't been able to talk to her now for over a week.

I was truly lost without her.

Chapter 8

TALKING TO MOLLY

I WASN'T SURE WHAT TO EXPECT when we did talk because I didn't know how she was emotionally. I wasn't even sure if she would talk to me. She may just need to sit with Maggie and cry, or she may need to talk to me and laugh a little. I knew I had to be supportive to whatever she needed. In the case that she didn't feel like talking to me, I asked Maggie to give her a kiss on the cheek, say it was from me and that I was thinking about her. Of course, Maggie agreed to do it, but she reassured me that Molly would talk to me that night. I just had to be sure that I was online.

I decided to be upbeat and fun when we talked. Then if she needed me to be sympathetic, I would be able to handle that. One of the qualities she loved the most about me was my ability to make her smile. Of course, I was glad to do that because she had such a great smile. I know I hadn't actually seen her smile yet, but we had such a strong connection, I could feel it. I knew she probably hadn't smiled at all that week, so I wanted to make sure I did that for her.

After a long day of waiting, it was finally time to talk to Molly! I was so excited to see her online, as part of me thought she wouldn't be. I didn't think I was that much of a priority to her yet. We chatted for a few minutes, and then she got silent. I didn't know what was wrong. After a few seconds, she started typing again, but it was Maggie. She came up behind Molly and gave her my kiss and it touched Molly so much that she started crying. Maggie said she would be a few minutes. When Molly came back, she told me I was the sweetest guy in the world and that she really needed something like that. I guess I made the right move?

She then apologized for not being able to meet me for dessert like we had planned. I made a joke about how I was really looking forward to a piece of pie because she always told me I ate too much sugar. Dental hygienists are always worried about teeth falling out. I think it's just a conspiracy to keep people from enjoying good food! I did make her laugh a little when I said that, so that was good. Then I told her not to worry about staying up there because I wasn't planning on going anywhere. We could see each other when she got back. At least now she had a laptop, so we could talk just as if she were home.

James would be in the hospital for a minimum of 6 weeks, which sounds like a big problem for my chances with Molly because she was going to stay up there the whole time. My friends told me I was crazy and that I should just tell her it was over if she didn't come home, but honestly I didn't agree with them at all. I have two lady friends, and if it were one of them in the hospital bed, I would be right there for them. Molly was actually a little intimidated by one of them because she isn't married, but I explained to her that she had to get over it as we were a package deal. She is family to me and always will be. If a girl can't understand that, then she can move on. How could I be that hypocritical and tell Molly she had to come home? I have always been a believer in treating others how you want to be treated. Typical "dating rules" would tell me to move on and find another girl, but there was nothing typical about my relationship with Molly. There was nothing actually wrong with me continuing to talk to her and seeing what happened. Some people may not agree with that decision, but we all have our critics in every decision we make.

Chapter 9

❧

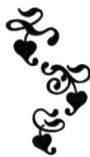

❧

HOCKEY TOURNAMENT

*T*HE 6-WEEK DELAY ACTUALLY COULDN'T have happened at a better time, as I was in the middle of planning a wheelchair hockey tournament. I did hate that Molly was going to miss the tournament, though. The timing would have worked out perfectly if we had had our first date as scheduled; I had the next weekend off, so we could have spent more time together and she could have met my parents (this has to be done early, being I live with them and can't drive due to my disability). The next weekend was our last hockey game before the tournament; Molly could have experienced that before being thrown into a tournament. An event like that can be a lot to take in for some-one who has never seen it. I know she would have loved to see me play, and I was looking forward to trying to impress her, but it was probably better that she couldn't be at the tournament as I didn't have much time to spend with her. Molly was very under-standing about my hockey program and would never stand in the way of it, but I would still feel bad if I wasn't able to devote as much time to her as she deserved.

Of course, Molly was really sad to be missing the tournament, but I tried to comfort her with telling her she was doing the right thing. Even though it wasn't what I wanted, it was right of her to stay there, and nobody can change my mind unless they have been alone in a hospital bed. Maggie was also going to visit her the weekend of my tournament, so I knew time would fly by for her. I told her I would still be able to email her at night before going to bed, but I couldn't chat online as I would be with the team or resting. When I got to the hotel, I found out that web service was $10 a day, so I wouldn't be able to email her either. I was able to send short emails on my cell phone, but it takes forever to really type much on there even with a keyboard.

On Thursday night after handling all the registrations for the teams and getting back to my room, I emailed Molly to let her know I had to use my phone and that my emails would be short and sweet. I told her so far everything was going well and that I would let her know how we did after our game on Friday.

Unfortunately, that would be the last email I sent Molly for a few days.

Chapter 10

❦

EMERGENCY ROOM

*E*VERYTHING STARTED OFF GREAT ON Friday. I went to the gym in the morning to make sure the facility was set up properly, then went back to the hotel for a radio interview promoting our tournament. I ate a good lunch because I knew it would be late getting back for supper after our games. The opening ceremonies were at 5:30 pm. There was another game before ours, so we would be playing at around 8:00 pm. We normally play at night, so this wouldn't be any different from our usual game day routine. I normally would eat a snack around 4:00 and arrive at the gym by 5:00 for a game at 7:00, so I didn't think this would be any different.

However, there was one issue I didn't account for. It is a lot of pressure coordinating an event and setting everything up, then participating in the event as well. Hockey is very demanding on the body at all levels, regardless of whether or not you are actually skating. When I first started playing, I was one of the naïve people who thought because I was just driving my chair, I could play all day. Ironically, I even found out that I couldn't play with a sprained ankle! In our game there is a lot of starting and stopping, which puts a lot of pressure on all parts of your body. You really have to be in the best possible shape to play wheelchair hockey.

In all the chaos of getting opening ceremonies ready, I forgot to eat my pregame snack, which is usually something high in energy and involves peanut butter, chocolate, or both. Bananas are also great, as the body digests them quickly into energy. I didn't realize how important this little snack was until I missed it. I also didn't realize that I had blood sugar issues!

After our game, I started to feel really nauseous. I didn't realize how empty I was during the game because adrenaline was keeping me going. When we finally made it to a restaurant, I ordered my meal but was unable to eat it. I asked my best friend to take me back to the hotel where I could relax and just drink some fluids. I knew I was dehydrated, so I was hoping that by slowly drinking fluids, I could settle my stomach and then try to eat something. However, that didn't work because as soon as my parents got in the room, I started vomiting. Everything I drank came right back up. The vomiting continued throughout the night, and I eventually had to go to the emergency room, which lucky for me, was right across the road from our hotel.

I'll never forget when I went in the room because I went right by the check-in tables to a lady I saw near a computer. She looked up to tell me to go the check-in area, but when she saw my face she said, "Whoa, you're sick, aren't you!" Normally, I would have been insulted because I like to think I look nice, but this was different. I had to get some fluids and get back to the hockey tournament! She immediately got me into one of those holding rooms in the emergency room, and they started getting me ready for an IV. Unfortunately, I was all dried up from being dehydrated and they had a hard time finding a vein. I swear they stabbed me 5 times in each hand!

When they finally got me hooked up, they did a bag of fluids, but also did a syringe of sugar water because their blood tests showed my blood sugar was really low. Of course, common sense could have told them that, as I hadn't eaten in approximately 18 hours and was up all night vomiting! I really wanted them to give me something for the nausea because then I believed I could eat, but they wanted to get my fluid and sugar up right then. They were very concerned about food taking too long to digest even if it stayed down. I didn't realize how serious the situation was, but apparently I was almost in trouble again like the year before. After that experience, I'll gladly let doctors do whatever they need to do.

Part of me believed that after they kept me a few hours, I would be good to go and would be back in the tournament. I knew I couldn't play our games Saturday, but felt I could get in the final games on Sunday. I really wanted to participate in those. The final games were being played in the RBC Center, home of the Carolina Hurricanes; playing in that facility would be a dream come true for me.

My goal was to be healthy enough for that, even if that meant staying in the hospital overnight.

Chapter 11

❦

HOSPITAL STAY

MY OVERNIGHT PLAN DIDN'T WORK out, how-
ever, because of the blood sugar issues. At first it was too low
because of the vomiting, then it was too high, which may have
been because of the shot of sugar water. That warranted testing
for diabetes; we have a history of that in our family, and it's fairly
common with my disability. I was going to be stuck in the hospital for a few more days.

I really hated being stuck in that room. Not only was I missing the tournament I'd worked so hard to set up, but I also felt
like I was letting both my team and the Hurricanes staff down.
The Carolina Hurricanes have been extremely supportive of my
program over the years. They helped me start it during my internship with the franchise, and to this day they are just an email

away when I need some help. Earlier in the year they even honored our team and me by letting me go on the ice and stand with the Hurricanes during the National Anthem! After all of their help, I wanted to show them a great tournament so they could see our sport at its best instead of just listening to me talk about it. I couldn't have asked for a better tournament, but having to miss it put me in a pretty bad mood in the hospital.

Needless to say, I missed my nightly emails to Molly. I didn't even check my own messages for about four days. When I finally checked it, I had one message from her just seeing how the tournament was going; she knew I would be busy and couldn't reply. Of course, the date on that email was 2 days ago, so I knew I was in trouble. After being stabbed so much for the IV, my hands didn't really feel like typing on a full size keyboard, much less a tiny phone keyboard, so I asked my best friend, Mickey, to email her just to let her know what happened.

At this point in our relationship, only a few people knew about Molly. I hadn't told my family yet because there really wasn't much to tell. Plus, I knew their reaction would be negative. They would say I was wasting time and talk about how dangerous it was to meet someone online. I wasn't ready to have that discussion yet since Molly and I hadn't even met. I did finally tell one of my sisters later during the summer after a family cookout at her house. They were talking about marriages and how long you should date before getting married. My sister said that I was going to be the one in the family who just showed up one day and announced to the family that I was married. I almost choked on my food! Then I just smiled and said, "No I won't be married, but I may get someone pregnant." Of course, they all laughed and moved on to the next topic. However, the next day I emailed my sister and told her about Molly. She was so shocked that she didn't respond or even talk to me for three days. I finally called her because I was about to go nuts to find out her reaction. She was really just surprised at how well I hid it, but my family doesn't often ask me about my relationships and that's not a topic I discuss openly.

So Mickey emailed Molly and told her that everything was fine, but I got a little overwhelmed and was in the hospital. That was all he told her! I had an email from her that afternoon; she was worried sick about me. She hated that she couldn't be with me, but then again it wouldn't be the best place for her to be introduced to my family. I really didn't want her there, anyway, as I couldn't have the first time we met be with me in a hospital bed. That wouldn't really look too well when you're trying to convince a woman to look past your disability and see that you are just like any other guy.

I finally convinced the doctors I wasn't diabetic and they let me go home after five days in the hospital. I was still a little queasy on my stomach and just tired from being sick, so I wasn't 100% when I went home. Molly became my nurse from far away as she was always checking on me to make sure I got my strength back. When we would chat online, she would even make me turn the computer off and go rest if we talked for over an hour.

Although she wasn't here, it was nice having someone making such a fuss over me, but that wasn't the best part.

Chapter 12

❦

MOLLY IS JEALOUS

*M*OLLY KNEW THAT DURING THE tournament we were going to take some of the younger guys out and flirt with some girls. Part of the joys of running the wheelchair hockey program is watching the confidence of our athletes grow. Even with my own issues concerning relationships or whatever, I will talk to just about anybody. It's especially easy when I have my teammates with me. When you are the one guy in a room in a wheelchair, people merely think it's great you're out of the house, so they won't really approach you. However, when you have a whole "pack" of guys in chairs, people get curious and will actually approach you to see if there is a disability convention or something. Most of the time they become intrigued when you tell them you're playing hockey against the best in the world. This is great because when new people find out you're an athlete, their entire perspective changes about you.

I have noticed too often in society that because I'm in a wheelchair, it is automatically assumed that I have mental disabilities as well. Whenever people find out we play a sport, it's like we are bought up to their level… where we should have been in the first place. I don't believe they're discriminating, I believe they just aren't educated. That is why part of our mission with our hockey program is to educate society on the abilities of disabled athletes. When you look at my relationship with Molly, we developed something because she wasn't afraid to ask questions, and I wasn't offended to answer them. Had I approached her with a negative attitude and forced her to treat me equally, she would have never talked to me. I was able to not only change her view on me, but on people with disabilities in general. She no longer had that fear of the unknown, which is why she was actually really mad at me when I didn't email her for those couple of days.

Molly felt certain that any other girl could fall for me as easily as she had, so her thought was that I'd met someone at the tournament and that that was it. She thought I was tired of waiting and had thrown her away like any other girl in order to move on to the next one. She always knew I was keeping my options open because I couldn't wait forever for her to make her decision, and she really thought I was gone. She felt horrible when she found out I was sick, but when she finally told me what she was thinking, I was actually flattered. Here I was, always skeptical that a girl could ever look past my wheelchair, and I had a gorgeous woman actually thinking I was a typical jerk! I was finally on the same playing field as all other men!

However, deep down, she knew better, and I was not a typical guy. We started complimenting each other by saying we were "abnormal." I'm looking for the amazing person to spend the rest of my life with; why would I want someone who is just like everyone else? Molly felt the same way. However, I did tease her for months about her insecurities about me leaving. It was my way to pay her back for the lingerie email!

Chapter 13

❧

PATIENCE MAKES THE HEART GROW FONDER

AS JAMES CONTINUED TO RECOVER in the hospital, Molly and I continued to talk every day. Her parents got her a hotel room and a rental car, so she was able to leave the hospital whenever she needed and didn't have to rely on James' parents. I'll never understand how her parents could afford that, and part of me wished they would tell her to come back home, but I was glad she didn't have to stay with James' family the whole time. I would never get to talk to her if that happened. As it was, it was almost like she was still at her house because I had my "morning coffee" email every day and then I would have one waiting for her when she got back to the hotel room in the evening, almost like she was at work. Then we would chat online at night for about two hours as always.

It was strange because I wasn't really concerned about her spending all this time with James. I guess it was because I knew it was just a matter of time before she would be home and I would get to meet her. That fear of not being good enough for her was gone. All I had to do was continue to be supportive and not try to rush her homecoming. I couldn't in good conscience steal a girl from a guy while he was injured, anyway. Plus, it just wouldn't look very good for me to force her to decide while he was injured. Knowing Molly, putting that pressure on her would have forced her away from me. It wasn't worth losing her just because I was being impatient. My father always said that "patience is a virtue." Of course, he used the adage to teach me how to fish when the fish weren't biting, but I thought it worked in this situation as well.

One major concern I did have was that Molly might be spending so much time at the hospital and she wasn't taking care of herself. I've noticed from my own time in the hospital that it can be very strenuous on families and friends when they stay in the room with you all the time. They don't eat good meals because it's so much more convenient to have a burger or some junk food, and their bodies become weak. I tried to watch out for Molly and asked her what she ate every day. To no surprise, most of the time she reported she'd had a burger and fries for supper. At the hotel, she would have the free breakfast, and while at the hospital she would eat a snack, if anything at all. Sometimes she would skip supper all together and have a bag of popcorn when she got back to her hotel room. I tried to get on her a little about that by telling her she would be in the hospital herself by the time James recovers, and then I'd have to wait even longer to meet her. Of course, I could only get so upset when she would say that she didn't eat because she wanted to get back to the hotel and take her shower, so she wouldn't be late talking to me. She really enjoyed our chat time; she said it kept her from having a nervous breakdown. She was really starting to miss home and was sick of being in the hospital all the time, even though she knew it was where she needed to be.

Fortunately, Molly's parents missed her too, so they came to visit her on weekends. Maggie also hitched a ride with them, which made me feel better. Of course, they had to go visit James, but they also got Molly out of the hospital. They would take her to eat real food, shop, or anything else fun that Molly wouldn't do while she was by herself. Maggie would also take her to the hotel pool or for a walk on the beach. Then she stayed in Molly's room, and they basically had little slumber parties like they'd had when they were kids. Molly's parents stayed in their own room to give the girls some time alone.

I absolutely loved their girl time because that meant they could talk about me! Molly had no friends up there besides those she and James went to visit, and Molly couldn't talk to them about the other man in her life. I've never had girls talk about me like that. While it was flattering, it could sometimes also be embarrassing. Every Monday after Maggie visited Molly, I would have an email from Maggie asking me questions about certain things

I had told Molly. Most of the time, these would be embarrassing moments from my childhood that I would tell Molly just to make her laugh. Normally, I would be upset with someone sharing my secrets, but Molly wasn't making fun of me. She was telling Maggie because she thought that my stories were sweet and adorable. Maggie actually told me that she was getting sick of hearing "how wonderful Jonathan is," but then she would immediately tell me how glad she was that I was making Molly so happy.

Finally, one weekend that Maggie didn't go visit, I got some good news. Molly's parents were visiting on that weekend as always, so during our chat Sunday night I asked Molly about her day. She told me they went out to eat (she knew I would worry about that) and that they took her rental car back to the dealership, which meant she wouldn't be there much longer! James' doctor told him that he would probably be able to go home at the end of the following week, so Molly would be able to just ride home with his family. There was no need for Molly's parents to come back up the next weekend to return the rental car and settle the hotel bill, so they took care of everything while they were visiting. Molly would just have to ride around with James' parents for a week, which was a little inconvenient, but not a serious problem.

We didn't talk much about how soon we could see each other after she got home. I knew it would be at least another week because she needed to rest, and their families were going to have a welcome home party for them. I didn't particularly care for the idea of their families doing that because it was just another thing to make it harder for Molly to leave that situation. Her mom was the only person in her family who knew about me, so the rest of the family didn't know any better. However, I knew it was something she needed to do just because it was right, so I encouraged her to attend. I knew Maggie was going to be there, so she would take care of Molly. I also knew that the party was mostly for James. He was more seriously injured in the accident, and his parents were hosting it. While Molly's friends were going to be glad to see her home, everyone knew she was away so long being a support system. James was the one fighting through a long recovery.

It's strange how a near-death experience will bring everyone out to see you. When I had pneumonia, I received over 200 get-well cards. It was amazing to see all the support from the community and from people I didn't even know. It was also funny to me because I got cards from people I haven't talked to in over five years; I don't even know how they knew I was sick. I assumed the same thing would happen for James. Of course, people would come in and hug Molly and say they were glad she was okay, but then all the attention would go to James and she would be left in the shadows. That sounds bad, but that was exactly where she wanted to be.

Molly knew she was ready to move on to something new. She just had to do the right thing and attend the party. The next day, she was going to have dinner with her family. They had invited James, but after that we could really start our relationship. Of course, I wasn't really excited about the family dinner, but the only thing I cared about was that Molly was finally coming home!

Chapter 14

❧

ANOTHER SETBACK

*T*HAT SUNDAY I SPENT THE day with my sister. I went over to her house, and we baked a cake. Sometimes we like to do that as our bonding time and, being she was one of the few who knew about Molly, I thought it was a good way for me to let some hours pass by. Not to mention I really like sweets! I didn't want to spend the day thinking of her having a family dinner with James still there. All I wanted was for it to hurry up and be nighttime so I could talk to Molly, and James would be back at his house.

I was watching television with my sister when I decided to check my email. I knew it would be about time for Molly to come home, so I wanted to see what the schedule was and when we could chat. After being gone so long, I wanted to give her plenty of time to clean her house or whatever she needed to in order to get settled back in. I travel a lot with my hockey team and know how you just need some time alone when you first get back home to relax and get re-acclimated to your surroundings. I was thinking she would say that she just got back home and she wanted to take a bath, straighten up the house a little, and just relax for an hour or so, then we could chat as usual. My assumption was way off, as the email caught me off guard.

Molly's brother was also in town for her homecoming, so her parents wanted to tell them some bad news while they were all together. While Molly was away, her mom's cancer had returned. There was a tumor in the same area on her back, and she would have to go through chemo treatment for the next six months. The tumor was surrounded by blood vessels, so it was too risky to do surgery and remove it. While I hated to hear the news, of course, I wasn't too surprised that the cancer had returned. One weekend when her parents came to visit, Molly said her mom was really tired and not feeling well. I have lost family members to the disease, so I knew fatigue was a symptom of cancer and the chemotherapy that goes with treating it.

As I read the email, I immediately started thinking about how I could be supportive of Molly in this difficult time, especially her first breakup with James came because he wasn't there for her. I can also pretty much guarantee that he cheated on her as well before they broke up, but she never actually admitted it to me. She would never talk bad about anyone, but I knew the type of guy and had no doubts. I would later find out from Maggie that I was right; he was your typical jackass.

Although I was getting impatient, I didn't want to be the guy who runs away because my fairy tale wasn't going as planned. Therefore, the first thing I decided to do was keep Molly a secret from those who didn't know about her. I didn't need all of their comments implying she was lying about the cancer and just didn't want to meet me, or that I was wasting my time with her. No, I still didn't know if she was really the girl in the photos I was falling in love with, but it didn't matter. The bottom line was that a friend of mine, who was a major part of my life, was hurting and she needed me to be there for her. The very least I could do was just be a little more patient.

 I'd waited my whole life for her; what was another 6 months?

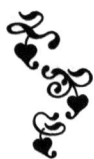

Chapter 15

MOLLY AND HER MOTHER

*M*OLLY ACTUALLY TRIED TO LET me out of our relationship when she told me about the cancer. She said that she couldn't ask me to wait that long for her, but she had to focus all her attention on her mom at that time. Of course, I didn't listen to her. What kind of guy would make a woman choose between him and her sick mother? If anything, the fact that she would give me up to help take care of her mom made me want her even more. I would never want a girl who would ignore a sick family member just to pursue her own desires.

Molly's mother was a hard-working, strong, independent woman. All of these characteristics rubbed off on Molly, which appealed to me. I've never been interested in the whiny, needy woman who believes she has to have a man in her life to survive.

To me, relationships have always been one of life's little bonuses. I believe they do enhance our lives, but they are not necessary for our survival. I don't want a woman who felt she would literally die without me. I want someone who can take care of herself, because how can she help me with my daily needs if she can't even take care of her own?

Because Molly had the same traits as her mother, she knew how stubborn her mom would be during the chemo treatments. Her mother was supposed to rest as much as possible at home after her treatments; therefore, she couldn't do the little chores around the house she normally did. She was a little obsessive about having a clean home and cooking meals, so Molly knew she would have to stay on top of these chores. Every afternoon Molly would go straight to her parents' house after work to cook supper and straighten up around the house. On the weekends she would do more, such as laundry and dusting. Molly knew she couldn't help her mother fight cancer, but she could help by making sure her mother had no excuse to avoid resting.

Every night after she finished her chores, Molly would go back to her house, and we would talk. She and I continued to grow closer by chatting online… about everything. She even answered my burning questions about the dentist. For example, both major toothpaste companies claim that dentists prefer their products, so I was curious as to which Molly preferred. I was a little disappointed to know that it really didn't make a difference. She said they basically do the same thing, so really I could use whichever tasted better to me. She did tell me I had to use the adult tarter control stuff and not the yummy stuff they give to children.

My other questions involved the tools that hygienists use. I wanted to know why they needed 10 different metal pick things that hurt (turns out there are different ones for different teeth), but my main interest was in the machines. For example, how strong is the suction machine they use? Can it pick up loose change off the floor like a vacuum? Also, what is the range of the squirt gun they use to rinse off your teeth? It turns out she didn't know because she never tested the power of the tools, so she couldn't answer those questions. However, she did say she would set me up an appointment one day and we could try it out! While I really was curious, I would have never done that. I just asked all those questions so that she would think about it and smile a little at work. It didn't hurt to know that she would be thinking about me at the same time! I loved being able to make Molly smile. She had a beautiful smile, which I think is a pre-requisite to being a hygienist.

Some people may believe such conversations are a waste of time, but I disagree. First of all, it is good to take an interest in your significant other's career. It shows that you care about their interests, and it gives you an opportunity to learn something new. Before Molly, I knew nothing about teeth other than they were used to chew food and you had to brush them. I had no idea why anyone would want to pursue a career in dental hygiene. It's a given that not all the mouths hygienists have their hands in are clean, and not everyone's breath smells good, so why put yourself through that? Molly explained to me that she didn't grow up wanting to be a hygienist all her life. She did, however, want to help people, and this was a good way to achieve that goal. She said that yes, sometimes staring at an infected mouth was a little gross, but it was extremely gratifying to know when that patient left the office, he was going to feel better. After she cleaned teeth, she was able to see a finished product, like a mechanic who builds a car. She knew that her job was helping people.

This conversation proved that Molly was caring and nurturing, important qualities I look for in women. The last thing I want is to waste time with a heartless woman.

Chapter 16

TEACHING HOCKEY TO MOLLY

WHILE I KNEW OUR CONVERSATIONS provided a good distraction from her worries with her mother, I did notice that Molly had started getting tired, so I eventually asked her if she would like to have our first date just to get her away from all the stress she had to deal with. It was not at all about me being in competition for her anymore. I wanted to take her out and let her smile some, although if she just needed a shoulder to cry on and an opportunity to let all her emotions out, I would be ready for that as well. I thought spending some time together would be a good break for her. She appreciated the offer but declined. She said that she knew after we met, she would never want to leave me. Then she worried that she would start to resent her mother for keeping her away from me. Of course, I couldn't let that happen, so I tried to explain that I wasn't the type of guy who had to see a girl every single day. I wasn't going anywhere. If we had our first date and didn't see each other again until after her mom was fully recovered, I was fine with that. She knew I would do whatever she needed and wasn't worried about me at all. She was worried about herself and her strong feelings for me. She didn't think she could see me and then go that long without seeing me again, so she wanted to wait to meet until her mother recovered.

I was so flattered when she told me that because I've never had a girl feel that strongly about me. Normally, I'm always wondering if they even like me or if they're just being nice; now I had this amazing girl thinking she could never get enough of me! This was all new territory to me, so I just agreed with her decision and decided to wait. Waiting wasn't really that hard because we did talk every day, and I knew she was too busy to see James as well. Not to mention it was almost the start of hockey season, so I would have plenty of distractions to help me pass the time until the chemo treatments were finished.

Hockey became a very important connection for Molly and me. She had seen my profile on the social networking site and was intrigued by my wheelchair hockey program. As we started talking about hockey, she immediately became a fan of the sport and of the Carolina Hurricanes. With everything the Hurricanes have done for me, you are pretty much forced to love the Hurricanes if you love me; they are more than just a team to me, they are family. It was also easy to make her fall in love with hockey because she thought all of the players were attractive! She would always try to tease me by saying whenever I took her to a game, one of the players would steal her away from me. Of course, I would answer that with the fact that they were already happily married.

Molly and I first started talking near the end of a season, so she was able to really get excited about the sport as the Hurricanes made a playoff run. We would watch every game on our respective televisions together, emailing each other our opinions on the team's performance during the intermissions. It almost felt like I was a coach because I would always have to boost her spirits. Hockey is a game that can completely change in a matter of seconds, so you are never really out of it until it's over. I remember in one of her first games, the Hurricanes were down 3-0 in the first intermission. She was disappointed and talked about not watching hockey anymore, that hockey could be my thing that I enjoyed alone. We didn't have to share every single interest as a couple. Everyone needs time alone occasionally.

However, I then explained to her that the game wasn't over. There were 40 minutes left in the game and the guys in the locker room certainly didn't believe it was over yet. If they could go out and play through the adversity, then it's our job as fans to stand behind them and believe in them. They were down 3-0, but they only needed to get three good shots on goal to be right back in the game. If you have ever seen a hockey game, you know it only takes a few seconds to get a shooting opportunity, and the Hurricanes had 40 minutes! I liked those odds! The Hurricanes ended up winning that game in overtime. From that moment on, Molly was hooked on hockey.

As the season ended, Molly even became interested in the off-season business of the sport. I majored in Business in college, so I admit the off-season is one of my favorite parts of hockey. Molly was out of town during most of the off-season because of her accident, but we still talked about it every day. It was a stressful time for us because we'd just had a good playoff run and had a few free agents that needed to be signed, one of which was one of our favorite players. Every night when we talked, one of the first questions she asked was if I had heard anything from the Hurricanes. It was so nice to finally have someone to talk hockey with!

Hockey also became an outlet for Molly while her mother was going through her chemo treatments. She wouldn't even watch the games at her parents' house. She finished her chores quickly so she could be at her own home to watch the game with no distractions. I was always glad to watch games with her because she truly fell in love with the game. I've noticed that when I introduce the game to people, their favorite part becomes the violence and the fighting. They fail to see the true beauty and skill involved in the game. In contrast, Molly hated the fighting and really appreciated the art of hockey. She learned to read plays and - the best part to me - was that when she had a question about a rule, she listened to my answer and then remembered it. I never had to repeat anything to her. We even got to the point

where we talked about coaching philosophies and team strategies. She truly impressed me with her newfound knowledge of
the game.

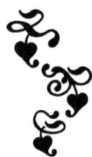

Chapter 17

❦

HOCKEY AND ME

*I*ALSO BEGAN TO DISCUSS IDEAS about my own hockey program with Molly. After my last tournament (when I spent the entire time in the hospital), I knew it was time to make some changes for my health. I had seriously considered retiring and focusing only on the management of the program. There is nothing I want more than to win our sport's championship, the Powerhockey Cup, but the game was getting to a point where it was too dangerous for me. In the past year, I had the horrible pneumonia experience, which caused me to miss a tournament, and the dehydration issues at the following tournament caused me to miss that event.

I knew that I couldn't continue playing at this pace and survive. It wasn't worth the risk. In the game that put me in the hospital, our opponents were a physically stronger team in faster chairs, and we lost 11-0. That doesn't mean they were better players, it just means they had better equipment at their disposal. I was starting to get disheartened with the game because it wouldn't matter what we did if other teams had assets like that. There needed to be some kind of standard in our game. Was it really worth it to me to put my life on the line to lose 11-0? I don't think so.

I talked to my vice president, who was also having the same concerns about the game and whether or not he should play anymore. The stress was just too much on both of us, as we were not only playing, we were also managing the business of the organization and trying to develop a winning hockey team for tournament play. We also had to spearhead all the fundraising activities in order to get a team to a tournament, all while training to actually play in the tournaments. My VP knew that he could no longer handle the stress of being a player. It was simply too draining on his body, and we both knew that his life was more important than his participation in a game.

He played goalie, which was a less mobile position, so he suggested I take over his duties there. Honestly, before our meeting, I had considered playing goal because I had about reached the highest level for me at a forward position. I was physically unable to stay with our competition, so the game became less fun for me. I had studied the game for 15 years and learned everything about the forward position, so the incentive to work hard was gone. I knew there was nothing left for me to do to get better. The only motivation I had for playing hockey was the physical benefits I felt from practicing. Hockey practice is a great form of physical therapy, so I wanted to continue to do the workouts in order to keep my body loose. With my disease, I cannot build muscle, but I do feel as though I can maintain what I have.

The other motivation I had was the responsibility to my teammates to be the best player I could be. I believed that by moving to goalie, I could help the team while rekindling my passion for the game by learning a new position. There is so much more to playing goal than stopping shots. You have to fully understand your positioning in the crease and not only stop the shot, but deflect the shot to an area where there won't be a rebound. You also have to know when to cover the puck and stop play or when to send it up to a teammate to start the offense. Without a doubt, it is the highest pressure position in sports and, while I was excited about the challenge, I was scared to death! It wasn't that I didn't believe I could learn the position, I was more afraid that if I couldn't actually do well at the position, my playing career would be over. I didn't want to kill myself playing forward, but I also knew I really wasn't ready to quit playing completely.

Even with everything Molly was going through with her mother, she helped me work through this trying time. I believe she actually enjoyed it because it was a nice break for her from the other stress in her life. She knew hockey was important to me, but we all know that in the grand scheme of things, my concerns about playing a position in a game were relatively insignificant. Yet Molly acted like it was the biggest decision in the world. She would always put the well being of those she cared about ahead of her own.

She addressed my goalie concerns by spending the next week trying to find me a goalie mask to wear. There was no doubt in her mind that I could play the position; her only concern was that I might get hit in the face with a shot or a stick. Of course, she didn't want my two front teeth to get knocked out again, but she didn't want my face to get bruised, either. She would always say that my smile and my honest face were her favorite parts about me, and she definitely wanted to protect that. However, I can't wear a typical hockey goalie mask because it is too heavy. My neck isn't strong enough to hold up the extra weight and be able to turn my head. That didn't stop Molly. She knew I wore protective glasses in games, so she started looking for different masks to cover just my mouth and nose. She emailed me all sorts of painter's masks and different things construction workers wore. I finally had to tell her to stop when she started sending softball face guards. I love softball, but I couldn't play hockey wearing a girl's mask! It took me a while, but I finally convinced her that I would be safe enough in a hat and my glasses.

Molly was truly excited about my taking the goalie position because her favorite professional player was a goalie. She couldn't wait to tell people she was dating a goalie, which was funny to me because I didn't even know we were dating! I loved to tease her when she made little comments like that without thinking. I believe that too often in our society we put too much emphasis on "dating titles." Have you looked at the steps to dating that people take today? First, they are "talking," then they are "hanging out," then there are other steps before they are officially "dating." I swear you need a guidebook to date in today's society! It is way too confusing for me.

All I knew was that Molly and I were falling in love, and I was just waiting for her to admit it.

Chapter 18

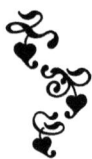

❧

HOCKEY TRANSITION

My fear of playing goalie wasn't the only problem with the transition. I wanted my vice president to stay involved with the team that he helped me build. The only way he could do that was to coach the team. That sounds like an easy decision because he knew the organization inside and out and also knew the direction we wanted to go as a program. In addition, as a former player, he had good knowledge of the game and knew how to push the other members of the team. As a general manager, he sounds like the perfect asset as a coach, but there was a small problem.

My father has done everything to help me start this program, which eventually resulted in his coaching the team. We had a volunteer coach at first, but he didn't have the time to dedicate to the program. When he stepped down, I asked Dad to be interim coach because he was great at teaching the fundamentals of driving the chair while controlling a ball with a stick. The fundamental skills of hockey are difficult enough on skates, so you can imagine the patience required to learn how to play the game in a wheelchair. Dad had started to become very stressed with all the issues off the court that go with coaching. Not only were we dealing with running the organization, but he also dealt with all the phone calls and emails from parents wondering what we could do to make their athlete better. Parents at every level of hockey tend to think their child can be the next Wayne Gretzky or something; it's hard for them to have the patience to let the coaches and veteran team members mold them into the best athlete they can be. Before letting your child play in a program, research the staff and the program itself. After that, the best thing you can do as a parent is trust that staff to do their job.

Dad did a good job getting the athletes ready to play hockey, but I knew his and my vice president's philosophies would be completely different. There was no way they could coach together. While they typically got along great, I knew it would eventually be a huge problem if they were co-coaches or even if one was the head coach and the other was the assistant. It wasn't that Dad did anything wrong, but by moving from coach to a more administrative position, he would be able to help me run the company and alleviate some of the stress on me. I also had to keep my VP involved in the team. The morale of the team would be very low if he wasn't there with us.

I was hoping Dad wouldn't be too upset. He wasn't being "fired," he was being moved to a different position. It was just too much on me to worry about the whole organization and all the individual needs of the players. While Dad would get the phone calls and emails, he would still talk with me about the situations to see what needed to be done. That was some extra stress we didn't need, so I honestly thought Dad would gladly give it up. I couldn't have been more wrong! Dad was very upset about losing the coaching job, which of course upset me because I couldn't understand why.

The night of that decision, I talked to Molly about it. I felt horrible because I certainly didn't want Dad to think I had fired him. After my two rounds in the hospital, people always told me that I needed to delegate more of the responsibilities. Successful Presidents have good people under them so they don't have to have their hands on every single thing that goes on in a business, and that is what I was trying to do. I knew my VP could handle the team and I could focus more on growing the organization by recruiting new players and starting new teams. Everything made perfect sense about the decision until Dad was upset about it. I felt evil. How could I put the organization's well-being ahead of my family? It was very frustrating.

Molly was able to work me through it, though. She explained to me that she knew I was one of the most caring people in the world and that I wouldn't make a decision that wasn't right for everyone. She knew I analyzed the decision from every view and thought about the big picture of the entire organization, not just our tournament team. She reminded me of the stress coaching was putting on Dad and me and that everyone was telling me to delegate. She knew that Dad was hurt at that moment about his transfer, but she also knew he would eventually warm up to his new job. She told me to be patient and that I had made the right decision, but it would take some time for everything to settle down. I admit I didn't really feel a lot better after our talk, but it was nice that she had that much confidence in me.

It probably doesn't come as a surprise that she was right, and now Dad enjoys his role as the assistant general manager.

Chapter 19

❦

CARING FOR MOLLY'S MOTHER

*D*URING HOCKEY TEAM DRAMA, I hardly realized that Molly's mother had already had three months of chemo treatments; Molly and I were halfway to being able to see each other - finally! More importantly, the doctors were confident that the chemo was working and Molly's mother would again survive cancer! She was getting weaker with all the treatments, but the tumor was getting smaller. Four months into the treatments, they even considered stopping because the tumor was almost completely gone, but the family decided to finish the six months in hopes that it would completely kill it and we would never have to go through this again.

Because of her treatment-related weakness, Molly's mother wasn't able to eat much, so the family basically force-fed her to keep her strength up. Even when she felt horrible, she would try her best to eat just to make Molly and her brother happy. It was a constant daily effort by the whole family to keep Mom alive; she really had no choice but to live. My family was the same way when I had pneumonia, so I understood how Molly's mother found her strength.

I was most impressed with how Molly's family took care of her mother. If one family member had a runny nose or any type of cough, they were not allowed to see her, and that included even Molly on a few occasions. Her mother's immune system was so compromised from the treatments that any type of bug could be deadly for her. I swear Molly would have taken the chemo treatments herself if she could! As her mother's strength declined, Molly would help her to the bathroom, get her dressed, and do whatever else she needed.

Occasionally, to get Molly's mother out of the house, the whole family would take her to the grocery store. Molly's brother and father would walk with her mother to help brace her just in case she started to fall, while Molly pushed the cart and got the supplies they needed. They wanted her mother to use one of the courtesy wheelchairs available at the store, but she didn't want to. She felt like those were for people who really needed it, as she thought about me. I told Molly to tell her that I take my chair everywhere I go, that I didn't need one in the store! Those are for her and she needed to use them. It wasn't like she was being lazy and didn't want to walk; it was a good idea to use it for her own safety and to ease the stress on those who cared about her.

Luckily, she never fell in the stores. However, she did fall at home one day while Molly was at work. Molly's dad was home and called Molly at the office immediately. I believe he called Molly just to have someone to talk to because he was more upset than her mother, who actually laughed and made a little joke before she would lay down to rest. Her blood pressure had dropped, and her legs just literally gave out on her. They talked to the doctor, who put her on bed rest for a couple of days. He didn't think there was any need to come in to the hospital because it was apparently a side effect of her chemotherapy.

I was relieved that everything was fine because one of my biggest fears was that I would have to meet Molly at her mother's funeral. I never told her that, but I did think about it to try and figure out how to handle the situation. How could I not be there to support her, but how could I let our first time meeting be at the saddest moment in her life? Luckily, the chemo was working, and it looked like I wouldn't have to worry about that.

One positive out of the whole situation was I was able to see how strong Molly was. When our relationship first started, we had concern about her being strong enough to be with me and take care of me. After watching her take care of her mother in her time of need, there was no doubt in my mind that she could handle the minor inconveniences that went with me. All I had to do was love her and make her "feel like the only woman in the world," as she said I did, and I would never have to worry about her leaving me. She truly was the type of girl that would be there for the proverbial long haul and wouldn't leave at the first sign of adversity. I often feared that when I met a girl, I would get sick and she would truly "see" my disability, causing her to leave because she couldn't handle it. I knew I would never have to worry about that with Molly, though. Our only concern was to get her mother healthy again. After that, we could meet and be together with no worries.

At least that's what I thought.

Chapter 20

❧

NEW PHONE

DURING THE CHEMOTHERAPY, I HONESTLY forgot about James. I don't know why, but I assumed that he just disappeared like he did the first time Molly's mother was sick. I hadn't heard about him at all, which I took as a good sign. Molly and I could talk about anything, which included what was going on with her and James. She knew from the beginning that my breaking point with people in general, not just women, was when they tried to hide things from me. Things always come back around and it was usually me sitting there looking stupid just because the girl wouldn't be honest with me. To me, that feeling is much worse than the feeling of rejection. Like I've said, I'll never hate a person for making a choice. It's their choice and doesn't make them a bad person, but they need to have the guts to be up front and tell me their decision themselves.

I always hated talking about James because he was able to do things I couldn't do with Molly. They weren't doing anything romantic, but at least he was actually able to see her. He knew where she lived, so he could just drop by to see her family and be able to spend some time with her. I would have done anything to be able to do that! As much as I hated to hear about him coming over or them going for a walk with Maggie and her boyfriend, it would have been even worse for Molly to try and hide it from me. I always respected her for being upfront about James. Realistically, she didn't owe me that. We weren't "officially" dating; we hadn't seen each other or even heard each other's voice. We knew we would eventually be more than an online connection, but at that point the only true "bond" between us was in our hearts. We weren't an item, and she wasn't cheating on me by spending time with James. If anything, she was cheating on him with me. After a couple of months without hearing anything about James, I thought he was gone. I knew Molly didn't have the time to go to the park or on their little afternoon "dates" because she was constantly taking care of her mother. I was confident that after Molly's mother recovered, there would be no more obstacles between us.

One night after we had been talking online for about an hour, I finally asked Molly if she had been able to get a new phone yet. Her phone was destroyed in the car accident, and it would be a while before she could break away from caring for her mother to go to the store for a new one. I learned then that James had bought himself a new phone and bought her one on his plan.

Of course, it took me a minute to calm down before I could talk to her about it, but she'd known I wouldn't be happy about it. James had told her he knew she would need it in case her family needed her, so he just bought it. He didn't ask if she wanted one or anything, he just showed up with it. She didn't feel she could tell him she would get her own phone and didn't want his, but I still didn't feel much better about it.

Normally, in situations like this with women, I'll just shut down and not show my true feelings, maybe because I'm always trying to preserve a friendship. However, it was different with Molly, and I believe that was mostly because I never had to actually see her. I could say what I needed to and not worry about the consequences. If she hated me afterwards, then I would lose her, but it would have been so much easier to move on than it would be if we worked together and saw each other every day. I believe people hold in their true feelings to prevent awkward confrontations. For example, in high school, you may wait until after a semester ends to break up with someone, so you won't have to see them in the same classes. Of course, if it's a mutual decision, that's not a problem, but if they cheated on you, the last thing you want is to see the person who broke your heart on a daily basis.

In my opinion, that was one of the greatest benefits of meeting someone online. Of course, with my hockey program, I can be found easily and have to be careful who I talk to, but it's so much easier to disappear and start over online. You can be yourself and let out your feelings. When Molly told me about her new phone, I let all the emotions out.

She didn't want to tell me and was actually hoping I would never ask about it. I had thought about not asking and just waiting on her to call me, but my hands were getting carpel tunnel typing 2 hours a night every single night, and I was also getting frustrated and a little impatient. I understood waiting until her mother recovered and was more than willing to do so, but I thought it was about time for a little upgrade in our relationship. We started off with emails, moved up to online chats, and now I really felt it was time for the phone calls.

After all, I had now waited almost eight months to meet her.

Chapter 21

FRUSTRATION

As YOU CAN IMAGINE, THE frustrations boiled over as soon as she told me about her new phone. Immediately, I wished I hadn't asked about the phone; it went back to something being hidden from me because she knew it would upset me. I then relaxed and told myself that this was a different situation and that I knew in my heart she was better than other girls in my past experiences. To try to lighten the mood a little, I asked her if something was wrong with that phone because there was no law that she couldn't use it to call me. Her answer pissed me off even more!

Molly said that she couldn't call me because then James would have my phone number. I told her that if he had half a brain he could look up my number through the hockey program. It's my choice whether or not to answer the call. She was actually worried that he would fuss at me or even find me to fight me. I wasn't worried at all because if anyone ever called me like that, I would call the police. I'm not ashamed of it. The police are here to protect us from crazy people. We pay taxes to make sure they are here when we need them. I don't have a male ego problem that says I have to fight for a girl with my fists. If I was dating someone who was calling another man, I would be mad at the girl I was dating, not the guy she called. I've never understood that and told Molly I wasn't going to do some daytime television talk show drama. If she wanted to call me, she could. I was not afraid at all of what he could do.

Her fear led me to tell her about another theory of why James was nice enough to buy her a phone. Cell phones are a form of electronic handcuffs that people use to keep up with others. By paying the bill, James was able to track every call and know plenty about Molly's conversations. He was also able to call her at any time; Molly had a guilt obligation to answer it because he was nice enough to buy the phone for her. It was really a perfect setup. Personally, I would never share a phone bill with a woman unless I was married. Needless to say, the phone conversation didn't come back up for a while. Molly knew I wasn't happy, but she also knew I would get over it. She told me the phone was going to be returned and she would get her own as soon as her mother's treatments were finished. That's all I could ask.

After that argument, we never discussed calling each other again.

I had said my thoughts, and she knew how I felt. There was no reason to hold a grudge because I knew she would call me when she was ready. I also didn't want to harass her everyday asking if James called or if she got a new phone yet. Common sense would have already told me the answer to those questions. The phone situation was a small wound in our relationship, but it would heal. Of course, if I kept picking at the scab, it could become infected and end up worse. I believe this happens a lot in relationships. People hold grudges over minor arguments and continue to bring them up at different times. Then the small arguments turn into huge problems for their relationships.

If you look at our argument about the phone, the truth came out. She defended her points and I defended mine. We listened to each other and understood both viewpoints. We then reached the compromise that Molly would get her own phone as soon as her mother was well and she had the time to go get it. Molly didn't want someone paying her own phone bill, anyway; she was a very independent woman. I was hurt that she hid the phone from me, but if I were in her position, I would have handled it the same way.

By talking about it, we were both able to understand each other's feelings and work through them. Molly and I had little arguments just like every other "couple," but we were always able to work through them. It wasn't easy for us because neither of us was particularly good at communicating our feelings, so it was a little adjustment having someone care for us as much as we cared for each other. We could tell by the mood of our online chats if one of us were upset about anything, even though when you asked what was wrong, the answer would always be "nothing." We knew not to push the other and that we would both talk when we were ready. However, sometimes I could get her to open up by saying, "Molly, sweetheart, I know something is wrong, but I can't make it better until you tell me what it is."

Chapter 22

❦

TESTING THE LIMITS OF PATIENCE

*T*HE GREATEST STRAIN ON OUR relationship came about a month after the phone argument. It was a great test for us, but it made our relationship the strongest it ever could be. I got an email from Molly one evening; it was very short, but she had to get something off her chest. She knew I didn't like things hidden from me, so she told me that James was still coming over for visits. I guess he just sat around her parents' house while she was taking care of them, but it still felt like he thought they were dating. Molly wasn't doing anything to make him think he wasn't welcome there, but she wasn't spending time with him like they were dating. He was just there. She knew I would be upset, so she said I didn't have to talk to her that night if I didn't want to. I was just supposed to let her know.

I was extremely upset. Here I was sitting here being patient and waiting forever for her, and he was still getting to see her. On top of the phone issue a month ago, it pushed me to a boiling point. I didn't know what to do, so I knew I needed some alone time to think about it. I replied to Molly's email and told her that I wasn't happy and to give me a day to get my thoughts together. I would talk to her again, just not that night. I couldn't. If I talked to her that night, I would have said something I'd regret and chase her out of my life completely. Although I wasn't happy with her at that moment, I knew I didn't want her gone forever.

Molly was really scared of my follow-up email because she knew she was going to get the "wrath of Jonathan," as she called it. She was always scared of the day when I would just blow up because I was always so nice and rarely had ill will toward others. She hoped that when I did blow up, it wouldn't be because of her; now she believed her biggest fear was coming true. In all honesty, she was close to being right. All the time I had put into our relationship and the patience I had while she was making her decision seemed worthless because he was still there. I was very frustrated.

The first thing I did was call my best friends to get their thoughts. Ironically, they did everything they could to calm me down. Normally, when a girl would hurt me, they would tell me to tell her to "go to hell" and move on to the next girl. For some reason they were different with Molly. They told me to calm down and talk to her. They knew she was very special and that I shouldn't treat her like past situations. These are the same people who told me four months ago to stop wasting my time with her and that she wasn't real! How did they turn on me and take her side? I knew in my heart they were right, though, and am so thankful they pointed me in the right direction.

Next, I sent Maggie a message and told her that Molly might need her support right now. I always did that when Molly was upset because I knew I couldn't be there for her and felt confident Maggie could take care of her for me. I told Maggie that Molly told me about James being around and that I wasn't happy about it. I did tell her that we would work through it and not to worry too much about it. I just needed a few days to get my thoughts together about it. Maggie replied to me and said that she already heard the news and hoped I would be all right because it really wasn't as bad as it sounded. James was just there. It wasn't like they were dating. Maggie was also over visiting one day when he was there and said that there was no connection between Molly and James. Maggie knew that I was the only person in Molly's heart, so she hoped I could get over being hurt. That made me feel better, but I was already to the point where I had made my decision.

I decided to lay out my feelings for Molly and, if she didn't accept it, then I was finished with her. I didn't want to put any more of my heart into something that may not ever happen. If James was always in her life, there would never be room for me. I worried that there would always be an excuse. She would never get over him and move on if she didn't do it now; it was time for James to go. I still didn't want to chat with her about this, so I sent her an email in order to get my thoughts out and clear with no distractions.

I started by saying I had calmed down and was going to try and get out my feelings about the whole situation. I was still upset, but she wasn't going to get the wrath of Jonathan. I was hurt, and this made it hard for me to completely trust her at the moment, but I could get there again. I explained that while the time getting to know her has been trying to my patience, it had also been one of the best times of my life. I had been patient the entire time with her decision making regarding me or James. However, I didn't want to stand in her way, nor did I want to wait around, either, so I did meet other women while I had been getting to know her. I told her from the beginning that it was a possibility that I would find someone else and she knew there was a risk in losing me while she was taking the time to make her decision. I always had to keep my options open.

In this message, though, I told her that no girl I met could begin to compare to her. She was everything I ever wanted, and I was willing to fight for her now, but she had to let me in the arena. It wasn't fair for James to be able to spend time with her if I couldn't. I was confident now that I was better for her, and I wanted my chance to prove it. I understood she wanted to wait until her mother recovered, and I was more than willing to wait for her then, but he had to stop coming over. If he didn't, then I needed to move on and see what else was out there for me.

I was really afraid of sending that message. While I wanted a romantic relationship with Molly, she really had become my best friend in this process. We all need that companionship and someone to talk to, and I'd grown accustomed to having Molly in my life. I didn't want to push her away, and I felt confident she would make the right decision.

I sent the email in the afternoon, so she would have it when she got home from work. It was part of our routine; I knew if she didn't have something waiting, she would have been upset, and I didn't want that to happen in front of her mother. I got a response from Molly at about 8:00 that night that said she was so glad to hear from me because she'd been very worried. She wanted to talk to me, but wanted to send it in an email as well because she wanted to be sure she covered everything. She said it was good news, or at least she hoped I thought it was good news. She also said that she was sorry she put me through all this heartache and that it wouldn't happen again.

After everything I had recently been through, I was really looking forward to hearing her "good news."

Chapter 23

❦

STARTING FRESH

I WAS FEELING PRETTY GOOD ABOUT myself and my chances after I read that message. I was so glad I hadn't made too much of an ass out of myself. I had never told a girl they had to make a choice between another guy and me, so I was new to the whole situation. I guess I handled it properly because two hours later, I got her confession.

The subject of the email said, "They say confession is good for the soul." In the first line she told me it was a long email, but to bear with her, as she couldn't hold this in any longer. She then apologized for the whole situation with James, not just recently, but everything. She said that I had been amazing and that she didn't deserve me. She said that she knew it was never going to work out with James when he came back in her life, but she was-scared of the unknown. She said that he was a great guy, but I no longer had to worry about him.

The last night when I couldn't talk to her, she called James and told him they needed to talk after work. They went out to a local fast food restaurant, but the sole purpose of this dinner was to break up with him completely. She told him that he couldn't come around her house any more, and he asked if I had something to do with the decision. She told him yes, and then he asked if I was jealous. Then she said that I wasn't, but they couldn't act like they were dating anymore because they weren't. He then said that he knew after the car accident that they were finished. He also knew what she was giving up by staying with him the whole time, and he could never repay her for that. James then told her that all he wanted was for her to be happy and he knew she wouldn't be happy with him. He told her he hoped that I was as good of a guy that she thought I was because she deserved the best. She told him thank you and that she knew I was the best already! He walked her to her car, gave her a last kiss, and told her he would always love her. Then he was out of our lives forever. Of course, as soon as Molly got in the car, she started crying, but I was really proud of her for waiting until she got in the car. Molly had such a great heart, so she cried a lot. She especially hated to hurt people even when she knew it was for the best.

After she left the breakup dinner, she went straight to her parents to check on her mom. Molly had told her dad where she was going, so he had told her mother when she got there. Her mother was lying in bed and asked Molly to get in bed with her and talk to her because she wanted to know the details.

Molly didn't know that her mother knew about the breakup; she just thought her mother could tell something was wrong. They had a great relationship, like life-long girlfriends, and had always been able to talk. Molly told her mother everything. She was the only family member who knew I existed at that point!

Molly crawled into bed, looked at her mother, and said, "Mom I need you do me a favor. I need you to stop inviting James over for family dinners or even to visit." Her mother then asked if this favor was because of me. Molly said that it was, but also that she and James were finished and they were never going to work it out. Then her mother asked what I had said about her decision and if we were dating now. At that moment Molly started crying.

Her mother asked what was wrong, and Molly said, "Mom I think I screwed up. I think I made Jonathan wait too long, and now I'm not even sure if he wants to be with me. He's very upset with me and I'm even worried that there may be someone else he's interested in. I don't know what to do."

Her mom then rose up in the bed, looked her in the eyes, and said, "Molly, that boy is crazy about you. He has waited this long just for a chance to meet you. Now you have ended a six-year relationship just because of him. Jonathan is available until he walks down the aisle with someone else. You can win him back before then. I'll never understand it, but there is something special between you two. Just be honest to yourself and with him, it will all work out."

I had always wanted Molly's mother to recover, but after reading that part of Molly's email, I wanted her to hurry up and recover, so I could give her a big hug and tell her thank you for everything. I always knew that Molly's mother was on my side, even though I was really scared of her parents. One of my greatest fears of being in a wheelchair and romantically involved with someone is the point where I ask the parents for permission to marry their daughter and I get the "how can you take care of my baby girl" question. I would be the same way if I were a parent. With limitations to how much money people with disabilities can make, it definitely becomes a concern. However, I knew I could handle this situation with Molly's parents if we ever got to that point by saying that Molly was a strong enough woman that she didn't need me to take care of her. Her strength and independence are two of the qualities I love the most about her.

I just needed a chance.

Chapter 24

❧

CONFESSION

I HAD ALREADY FORGIVEN MOLLY, BUT there was more to the message. Molly said, "All that being said, Jonathan, you said that you would fight for me if I would just let you in the arena. Well here's my confession. The truth is that you are the only person in that arena. It has always been you since we first started talking. I was too scared to admit it and I tried to hide in the past. I'm not sure what will happen between us, but I am sure that I want to pursue a relationship with you to see where we end up. I still have to take care of my mom until she recovers, so we will have to wait a little longer. However, after that, I am all yours. That is, if you still want me. I am truly sorry I made you wait this long and I am sorry that I hurt you. I hope that you can forgive me because I really think we will be great together. Please respond to this because my nerves are killing me! I really hope we can chat tonight too!"

For the first time in my life, I was speechless. I was so happy, I couldn't even react to what she said. I just sat there and stared at my computer for what had to be five minutes. I couldn't believe it was finally going to happen. When I first started falling for Molly, I honestly just wanted a date to see what would happen and, in the back of my mind, I always thought she would go back to James after meeting me. I was just feeling good that I actually had a girl get to the point where she wanted to meet me. I seriously thought she would be a building block to my confidence to help me pursue other women in the future without the fear of rejection. You can imagine my surprise when she actually got rid of James and wanted to be with me.

More importantly to me, however, was the fact that James was finally out of her life. From the beginning, I knew he wasn't right for her because he didn't appreciate her. He ran through the same old motions that so many other guys do with their girlfriends. Too often I see girls get trapped in these relationships, and I didn't want the same to happen with her. Molly wasn't a typical girl, so she needed an extraordinary guy to truly give her the happiness she deserved. Was I that guy? I don't know, and, yes, I had my doubts, but the bottom line was I wanted to show her she didn't have to settle for him. She deserved the best. I didn't know if that was me, but I knew for a fact it wasn't James.

It was a strange situation for me because I've always been good at the flirting and the chase of a girl, but I didn't know what to do when I actually caught one! Molly wasn't just any girl either; she was the woman of my dreams. She was true angel who just popped into my life. I was finally able to gain a bit of composure and send her a response. I wanted to stay cool and relaxed in my reply, but of course that didn't happen and she would have been able to see right through it, anyway!

In my email I said, "Wow! I really don't know what to say. I've never had everything I ever wanted in my life to just get laid out in front of me. We definitely have to talk tonight! Of course, I still want you. Your mom is right. I am crazy about you and that won't ever change. You are definitely forgiven and I know that I never have to worry about that again now that he is gone. Wow Molly I am just so excited! I'll be online at our normal time, so we can chat. I can't tell you how much I've missed you over these past 2 days. Talk to you soon!"

So, it was official! I guess I now had a girlfriend. Of course, I still hadn't actually seen her or heard her voice, but the connection was definitely there. It was just a matter of time before we took care of the other minor details. Until then, we were going to enjoy talking to each other as we always had. There was no longer any competition between James and me, and I stopped worrying about searching for other girls. The biggest problem we had to face now was the waiting. We also had to tell our families. Well, Molly had to tell hers before I told mine because she had to explain why James wasn't coming over anymore. She also had to tell her brother, so he wouldn't invite James over when he came to visit the family. I was lucky in that I could still keep it quiet; my parents didn't have to know until after our first date and before she came to my house. If I were able to live in my own place and take care of myself, my parents wouldn't know about a girl until I was ready for them to meet her. I was handling this situation in the same way. Any other guy or girl would have done the same thing. All right, so I had commitment issues as well and was just afraid to admit to my parents that I had met someone. My parents knew enough about me. I can't even use the bathroom without them knowing, so I think I deserved a little something to keep to myself.

Chapter 25

🌱

MOLLY'S FAMILY

AFTER MOLLY'S CONFESSION, NOTHING ACTUAL-LY changed. We had really been together this whole time, but we were just too scared to admit it. We even decided that our "anniversary" would not be the date we made things "official," but the date she first emailed me. I always used February 27th as our anniversary, anyway, because that was when she came into my life. I didn't need a title because to me our relationship started that day; we just decided to move the relationship to different levels as we got to know each other. February 27th is also my best friend's birthday, so it was really easy to remember. Trust me, it means a lot to a girl if you can remember the first day you ever talked to her. Any guy can remember the first kiss, first date, wedding, etc., but to remember the exact moment when that special person comes into your life means the world to her.

It was fall and nearing the holidays. This was a little tough for us because in a perfect world, we would have been able to spend our first holidays together. A majority of Molly's family lived in other states, so their Thanksgiving and Christmas celebrations were normally a small gathering of her immediate family. Her brother's girlfriend would come, too. This was the first year James wouldn't be there, so Molly had to tell her brother not to ask about him.

When she first told him they broke up, her brother wasn't surprised. He said, "Molly, we all knew things were different at the party after your accident. We knew it was just a matter of time. So, is there someone else?" Of course, that was the perfect opportunity to tell him about me. Molly and I were also alike in that we were very private about our personal lives, but if you ask the right questions, we won't lie to you. Lucky for me, nobody ever asked me if I was seeing someone. Some of my friends are probably mad that they are finding out about Molly while reading our story, but they never asked, so they only have themselves to blame.

When Molly started telling her brother about me, she started off saying that I was 28, had a job, a degree, etc – the familiar info you normally tell a family member about a new relationship. As he was about to ask for more information, their dad came into the room and asked him to help with some yard work. Her brother told Molly that the discussion wasn't over and that they would talk later. While he was there, her brother and dad also changed the oil in her car and gave it a quick look to make sure nothing was wrong with it. Her car was old and had high mileage, so they liked to take care of it for her. It was also some good "bonding" time for her brother and dad.

When Molly's brother came back into the house, it was time for supper. Molly had cooked the meal, and afterward, she and her brother would clean the kitchen and put away the dishes. Their parents would then go to their room so their mother could rest, so that was when the conversation about me would continue. Her mother hated to go to the room because she wanted to spend time with her kids, but they forced her to go rest. Her brother really just wanted some alone time to find out more about me.

He started off asking why I wasn't there today because he would have loved to talk to me while working on her car and tell me the truth about Molly. She laughed and said that not only would I not believe anything he said because I was a little brother and know all the tricks about how to get rid of our sisters' boyfriends, but I also wouldn't go out and work on the car. He then asked if I was a prissy boy afraid to get my hands dirty. Molly told him about my disability.

I was nervous about this, so when Molly told me, I asked her to describe his reaction for me. I had to know whether or not I had to sell myself to him as a good guy for his sister or if I had to get him to look past the disability as well. There are definitely different strategies there. Molly had almost eight months to get used to my disability before we met, but her family didn't. They were going to be protective of her until their fear of the unknown was gone, so I had to plan for that situation. The Americans with Disabilities Act cannot do anything for you in matters of the heart. There are no laws forcing a family to approve of you dating their daughter. You have to be the mature, open-minded, and over all good person in order to make them fall in love with you as their daughter did. Being defensive and belligerent won't get you anywhere in this situation. Would it help me to be mad because their house didn't have a ramp? No!

Luckily, it turned out that Molly was my biggest supporter and she basically "sold" me to her brother while they were talking. When she first told him I was in a wheelchair, he asked her if she knew what she was doing because they had never known anyone with a disability. She then told him how good I was about answering her questions and that we had talked in detail about what all I needed help with during the day. She admitted that she was nervous at first, but I helped her through it. She then told him how I didn't let my disability get in my way at all and told him about the wheelchair hockey program. That is when his eyes lit up. She had done it. She made him see past the wheelchair already to see me. He couldn't wait to meet me because he wanted to be a friend. He didn't care if I was dating his sister or not; he just wanted to meet this guy Molly thought was so great.

He then asked her how long I have been in the picture and she told him since February. He was shocked! Not only because she kept me a secret for so long, but that I was still there. He asked her what was wrong with me because he never knew a guy who would stay around that long without trying to get a girl in bed, and I didn't even have Molly's phone number. At that moment she bowed her head, started to cry, and muttered, "I honestly don't know why he's so good to me, but he is. He would wait forever for me and I don't understand why." Her brother then lifted her chin, wiped the tears away with his thumb, looked her in the eye and said, "Because, Molly, you finally found someone who knows how wonderful you are, and I am so happy for you."

At that point I had two thirds of the family supporting me. Her mom loved me already and her brother was becoming a fan. Maggie and I had become friends throughout this whole process, so I knew she approved of me. Now I just had to worry about Molly's dad. I knew from my own father that although he may seem nice, fathers are very protective of their baby girls. Molly's dad wasn't any different, even though she said he would love me because I made her happy and that's all he cared about. I trusted Molly and believed he would approve of me eventually, but I still wasn't going to be left in the room with him alone; she'd have to stay in there so I could hide behind her! We didn't have to worry about that meeting for a while though as Molly's mother still had treatments to take care of.

However, I knew the day I met the family would be coming soon.

Chapter 26

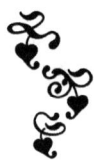

DISNEY WORLD

*T*HE WEEK AFTER THANKSGIVING, MY parents took me to Disney World for Christmas. My sisters were both born in Florida, and we try to go back occasionally. I love it because it's not so cold in the winter! I also absolutely love Disney World. Molly always said I was a big kid, so she wasn't surprised when I told her what I was getting for Christmas. To me, Disney is the only place where you can always act like a kid and have a good time without worrying about what everyone else is thinking. I believe life can be a balance of stepping up to your responsibilities and enjoying being alive. It's okay to be a kid sometimes!

I also really enjoy the creativity involved in making the animated movies. Imagine drawing a character whose image is ingrained into the minds of people for years! You can't do that with reality television. I bet that most people can't name two winners of a reality series, but they can most definitely name two Disney characters. I use to tell my parents that I was going to move to Orlando and marry Jasmine, from the Disney movie Aladdin. I actually met her on that trip and told her that she was my favorite part of Disney World. I think I made her blush a little! Of course, I had to send a picture with her to Molly. She was so jealous! I even sent her one with Jasmine giving me a hug, but it looked like she was kissing me. That really pissed her off. I thought it was hilarious! It wouldn't have been a problem if Molly had made up her mind earlier and she could have gone on the trip with me, so I had to have some fun with her.

I tried to take as many pictures as possible for my own memories of the trip, but also because Molly was stuck at home and I wanted to share some of it with her. She really enjoyed the Christmas season, as do I, so I wanted to get pictures of all the decorations for her at Disney World. I knew that they wouldn't have many Christmas decorations at her house because her mother wasn't up to it, so I decided her present from me would be a slide show of all the Christmas decorations. I didn't have her actual address, so I couldn't send her a gift, but I still wanted to share the Christmas Spirit with her just to try and cheer her up. I wanted to send her an actual gift, but of course she wanted to wait and do presents when we were finally able to see each other. We were just going to have to skip gifts this year.

Maggie and I had our own ways of sneaking around Molly's wishes, though, in that she would always drop by with flowers or Molly's favorite candy and say they were from me. I know I owed her over $100, but she never asked for a dime. All she cared about was that I was making her best friend the happiest she had ever been. Molly's mother even helped us out by giving Maggie the spare keys to Molly's house and car. While I was in Florida, Maggie left candy in Molly's house the first night I was gone, and she left flowers in Molly's car on the day before I came home. Molly actually got mad at Maggie and her mother for helping me out saying that I didn't need any help from them. I had already stolen her heart.

Molly had a trick or two up her sleeve as well. When I returned home, it was already mid-December, so my family was questioning whether or not to get a Christmas tree. The tree is my favorite part of Christmas, so I really wanted one, but I didn't feel right asking for it after they had spent all that money on my trip. It was also a lot of work for really only 2 weeks of display because we are old-fashioned and get a real tree. Molly went ballistic when I told her and she told me to do everything I could to get a tree. I thought she just wanted me to have a tree because she knew I loved them, but I found out the real reason about a week later.

My mom stopped by the post office on her way home from work one day. There was a box waiting for me, and she was curious as to who sent me a package. On the return address, Molly's friend had put her initials and Molly's, which tipped me off that it was something from Molly. I had no clue what it was, so I asked my nurse aide to help me open it, and Mom had to give us some privacy. She was about to go crazy because she didn't know who was sending me packages! My aide knew about Molly because I talked to him about her. I don't have a brother, so advice from an older male about dating was really appreciated. I wasn't expecting the gift to contain anything dirty or inappropriate, but I did want a moment to myself to enjoy it without all the questions from my mom.

I'm so glad I got that moment because there was a really nice letter inside the package that I still have put away. It was just so nice to know that I made her feel that special. The gift was small but meaningful. Her friend had found a Christmas tree ornament dealer at a local flea market, and she found a Carolina Hurricanes ornament. She bought one for Molly, so Molly asked her to pick one up for me because she knew I would love it. Molly gave her friend some extra money and also asked her to get me an ornament of a Golden Retriever if she could find one; I own a Golden, and she loved him so much. Sometimes I thought she was just using me to get to my dog! Finally, because of my sweet tooth, she put a tub of cotton candy in the box. I think Molly knew me better than I knew myself!

Molly also had done such a good job selling me and the hockey program to her friend that her friend put a separate card in the package with a $50 donation to the hockey program! Her card was also very nice, thanking me for making "our mutual friend" so happy and that she was so glad we found each other. She even used a Disney check with Aladdin and Jasmine on it.

After receiving her gift, I had to tell my mom about her. It was actually easier than I thought because my mom knows I'm a flirt, and she just thought another girl was being nice to me. She did ask if Molly had a boyfriend, and I just answered with "not anymore" because James was out of the picture. That was all the information my mom really needed to know at this point. She didn't need to know all the details of our relationship at that moment.

I didn't want to tell her just yet that the gift was from her future daughter-in-law.

Chapter 27

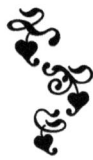

❧

CHRISTMAS

MOLLY AND I HAD DISCUSSED waiting until we met to start doing the gifts, which was fine. She also told Maggie because I tried to get an address from her, and she wouldn't give it to me! After I received my Christmas present, I thought, "Hey I can use the return address and still surprise her with a gift before Christmas." I really wanted to give her something even though she would have been mad at me for not respecting her wishes to wait until we met. If you look back at her year, it was horrible, so she really needed a present at Christmas just to cheer her up. However, she must have read my mind because the return address was her friend's address, and I couldn't send anything.

It turned out that all Molly wanted for Christmas was for me to be available to talk to her. We were able to spend Christmas Eve, Christmas Night, and New Year's Eve together chatting online. I know it sounds strange, but it was great sharing those holidays with her even though we weren't physically together. Holidays are a great time to be with family, but it's also tough if you are single because you wish you had that significant other like everyone else. Material gifts are great but are only a temporary fill to the loneliness and empty feeling. Even if you can't actually spend that day with your special person, a phone call, text message, email, card, etc., to show they are thinking about you means the world.

During this time, I started to understand how military families handled being separated on the holidays. They are halfway around the world, defending our freedom, and all they get is a few pictures emailed to them of their kids opening presents. Still, small gifts like that are why so many of our soldiers make it home. They know there are people here who love them even if they can't see them. I had the same feeling during that holiday season with Molly. Although I couldn't physically see her, that Christmas was one of my all-time best Christmases because I was able to spend it with her. As always, she was the last person I talked to on Christmas Eve and she still took the time to email me on Christmas morning before she went into the living room with her family. After we both spent the day with our families, we were back online Christmas night talking about our day. I'll never forget my first Christmas with Molly.

I was also really proud of Molly's brother on that Christmas Day because he helped make it special for the family. He knew that his parents couldn't go out and buy presents with his mother's illness, and he also knew that Molly wouldn't take the time to do it because she was so busy caring for her mother. He lived over 100 miles away and couldn't come over during the week to help take care of their mother. So to make Christmas a little extra special for them, he bought presents for everyone and placed them under the tree before everyone got up Christmas morning. Maggie also made Molly go shopping with her one day to get her brother a video game he wanted. They didn't have much, but I loved how they wanted to make sure everyone had a good Christmas.

Molly and her brother also gave their parents some money with the stipulation that they use it to take a trip after the chemo treatments were finished. They were hoping their parents would use it as a romantic weekend and just go somewhere together, but their parents wanted to do a family road trip. They wanted to drive to Oklahoma to pick up Molly's grandmother, who lived in West Virginia but stayed with family elsewhere during the winter months. She normally stayed with Molly's parents, but she couldn't this year because Molly's family had to take care of Molly's mother. This year she stayed with other relatives in Oklahoma, but she wanted to come back to stay with Molly's parents as she always had. Molly's mother also wanted her there as she rarely got to see her since she lived in West Virginia. She was missing their time together.

They wanted to leave as soon as the chemo treatments were over, so that meant Molly and I would have to wait another week to meet. She wasn't happy about it and didn't want to go, but I told her I could wait another week and wasn't going anywhere. Her mother would have just finished her second battle with cancer and she deserved this trip with all of her family. Molly and I could give her that and wait a little longer to "officially" start our relationship. Besides, it was December, and the treatments weren't over until the end of February (best case scenario), so one more week wasn't going to kill us.

We couldn't have imagined what was ahead.

Chapter 28

❧

MAKING PLANS

THE NEXT TWO MONTHS LITERALLY flew by. With James out of the picture, Molly and I were able to talk about more relationship-related topics and our future together. This was all new to me. We had already passed the sex talks a while back when Molly had her questions about my disability, but now we had started talking about having children. At first, it was whether or not we wanted a family in the future (yes). Then we discussed when we would want this family. Molly was only 23, so she wasn't sure if she was ready to have kids immediately. I really had no opinion because I didn't even know if I would be able to have children. I have talked to doctors before about the possibilities of me having a kid, and the only way to answer it was for me to give them a sperm sample. I decided to wait until I had a wife to help me out with that. I mean, really, can you hear that conversation with my parents? "Mom, Dad, I want to see if I can have children, can you help me get a sample for the doctor?" No thanks!

After talking to the doctors earlier in my life, I knew that if I were to get someone pregnant, it would definitely be a gift from God because my chances were less than other guys. Molly knew this, so when we talked about it, she said that if we happened to get pregnant, she would have the baby with me. Of course, that was the answer I wanted, but ultimately it was her body and her choice. Let's face the reality of it, I am in no position to raise a child on my own, so she had to want it. However, hearing her say she would have a child with me basically gave her the little bit of my heart she hadn't stolen yet.

As we continued to discuss our lives together, marriage came up. I am the first grandson in my family and am supposed to inherit my grandmother's engagement ring. I would like to give it to my future wife one day but also understood if she wanted a new ring that would be truly her own. That subject came up because I was afraid that my grandmother's ring had been lost one day. My grandmother had had an emergency, and the ring was misplaced. It was found the next day, but it was a little upsetting to me.

When I talked to Molly about it, she said she would love to wear my grandmother's ring if I thought she was worthy enough. I said that was good to know because I really didn't want to spend all that money on a new ring when I had a perfectly good ring that would remind us of a marriage that lasted over 60 years. Then Molly asked me if I was proposing, but I quickly answered with, "Molly. I don't even have your phone number!" She laughed and said as soon as she got home from her family road trip she was going to call me, so I would finally shut up about "our first phone call." Then we could go on our date and go shopping for her a new phone.

Chapter 29

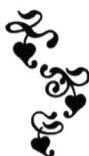

❦

THE BENEFIT

*T*HE DAY ARRIVED FOR MOLLY'S family trip. Her mother had beaten cancer for the second time, and we were all set up to meet. We had to wait just one more week, and it seemed like everything was finally going our way. The week was going to go by fast because I had a fundraiser for my hockey program on Tuesday night, and I had a lot of planning involved in making the event happen.

I come from a small town, and people my age always say there is nothing to do here, so they travel to other communities on weekends. At least that is always the excuse of why they can't come to my hockey team's games on Saturdays. Personally, I think they just don't want to come because they'd rather go out drinking, and we can't serve alcohol at our games. It goes back to the girls I'd try to date who didn't want to be honest with me because they figured I'd be disappointed. People didn't come to my games because they don't think the games will entertain them, but they didn't want to tell me that. They would rather spend the $5.00 admission on a beer instead of using it to make a difference in someone's life. However, that's their own choice and I'm not bitter about it.

I use obstacles like that as a challenge. I know a lot of people in the demographic from age 20-30, and if they don't want to watch hockey, then I would provide them with another form of entertainment to try and get them to support my program.

I decided to have a benefit rock concert in my community. I found a great local band, Airiel Down, and looked them up on a social networking site. It worked to find Molly, so I wanted to see if it would work for this as well. I sent the band an email. They absolutely loved our organization's mission and wanted to help us; I just needed to find them a facility, and they would be there. They also said they appreciated my professionalism in my request, as they get many requests daily from people wanting a donation of some kind. I felt good about that because I always want to be professional and a good businessman.

My colleagues in the hockey organization wanted us to have the concert away from my community in a market where the band was more well-known. However, I always had faith in my community that if I provided the right opportunities, they would come out and support me and the program. Not everyone likes sporting events, so I wanted to give this opportunity to my community. Plus, the theatre where we had the event was a great facility for the right price. We wouldn't find another venue like that for such a good deal.

I believe we did everything right. People said they leave the area on weekends, which is why they never came to our games, so I decided to have the concert during the week. It was a Tuesday night, so there were no church activities, and the college kids normally went clubbing on Thursday nights. We advertised the concert to all colleges, high schools, nightclubs, local businesses, and we even had a story in the local newspaper. I knew in my heart that we were going to sell out and have one of the largest fundraisers in our history!

However, as my luck would have it, a winter storm hit my town on the night of the concert. It wasn't too bad and schools weren't even delayed the next morning, but it was cold enough that I feared people wouldn't come out. Ironically, all my teammates and their families made it when cold weather and ice can be tough on people with disabilities. And that was about it for attendees. We had around 50 spectators when we were hoping for 500. Instead of making $5,000 on the fundraiser, we ended up losing $150 that night.

While the concert itself was amazing and all my teammates really enjoyed it, I was very disappointed. My family and friends knew it, so they tried to console me by blaming the weather, saying that nobody was coming out in the ice and that I couldn't do anything about it. They said I did everything right, and that sometimes these things just happen when you do events. I felt better until the drive home when I noticed that all the bar parking lots were full. People were willing to drive out in the ice to get drunk; why couldn't they come see our show?

I was really disheartened with my community because it just didn't add up. All I could think about was hearing from people who had said they'd come to something during the week, just not a game on the weekend, letting me down again. I wished they'd been honest with me and said they didn't want to help our program instead of letting me put all that time and effort into this event. I had done everything they asked by providing something other than a hockey game and by having it during the week when they were in town. The show was even over by 8:30, so they still had time go out and have a few drinks if they wanted. I didn't understand and never will.

That's not all I wouldn't fully understand.

৩

Chapter 30

TRAGEDY

IDID HAVE AN EMAIL WAITING from Molly when I got home; she wanted to know how the concert had gone. We couldn't chat because she was spending time with her family, but she wanted me to know she was thinking about me. Like me, she thought the show was going to be great, so she was very sad when I told her what happened. She was worried about me, so she had Maggie check on me the next day in case she couldn't email me herself. I then got an email pep talk later that night from Molly. She had a real knack for making me feel better. She always said I made her feel like a queen, like she was the only girl in the world. She always made me feel that special as well, although I'd never get to tell her.

I didn't know it at the time, but that little pep talk would be the last email I ever received from Molly. I responded to it, but it was the end of the week, and I wasn't expecting a response because they were supposed to be leaving on Thursday and be home late Friday night. We were going to have our first date the following week, then she would meet my parents the very next weekend. Our first date was really just a formality; we were ready to do the whole relationship thing.

I still hadn't heard from Molly by Saturday night and was starting to get worried. I was scared that there was another accident and that our meeting would be postponed yet again. I didn't want to worry Maggie yet, so I was going to wait until Sunday to email her. However, Sunday morning I had a message waiting from Maggie. Actually, it was from Maggie's mother because Maggie was too upset to send me a message herself.

There had been an accident, and it was a lot worse than the last one. I never got the details, but when Molly's family was driving home, their van lost control. There were no survivors. Molly, her parents, her brother, and her grandmother all died in the crash. She was gone and our little fairy tale was over.

At first, I refused to believe it. I went through all the stages of depression: anger, denial, and eventual acceptance. In the end, all I knew was that I was in love with a wonderful person, and I never had the chance to tell her. Her friends would later tell me that she knew and that she loved me with all her heart. She couldn't wait to meet me so that we could share our lives together. It was strange to build such a strong relationship with a stranger on-line, but I have no regrets.

She was an answer to my prayers and I truly believe that my angel had earned her wings.

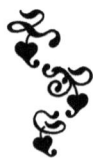

Chapter 31

TO THE SKEPTICS…

WAS MOLLY REAL? EVERY PERSON who hears about our story will have a different opinion. Trust me, for a while I had my doubts as well. I went through every scenario while working through my grief. I was most frustrated because I couldn't find any information on the accident. I waited to hear from Maggie, but she was having an extremely tough time dealing with Molly's death and wouldn't respond to anything. I emailed Molly's other friend who sent the Christmas present to see if she could locate any information. All I got out of her was that the family had a quick funeral service and burial. The bodies wouldn't be sent back home or anything, so not only would I never meet Molly, but I would never even have closure by being able to visit her grave.

The anger started setting in because the information they gave me wasn't good enough. How could a wreck that killed five people not be on the news or at least in a local newspaper? I looked online at all the newspapers for cities that would have been on their route home and couldn't find anything. I even had friends in the court systems and police departments do a search to find any information they could on the accident. We couldn't find anything anywhere.

My mind started to wonder if this whole year had been a scam. Was Molly real? I didn't have an address on her because she wouldn't let me mail any gifts. I didn't have a phone number because hers was busted in the first accident. I didn't even know where she worked because I really never bothered asking what dentist office employed her. I did know what city she lived in, but she rented a place and she would be hard to trace. It just didn't add up how she could just disappear like that.

During my investigation into Molly's death, I'm ashamed to say I took out my rage on her friends. I actually accused them of being Molly and that the whole thing was just a dirty trick. Fortunately, they realized I was hurting, and Maggie and I are still friends. I talk to her weekly, and we both have been able to help each other deal with the loss of our Molly. Maggie has even exposed more of Molly's secrets to me, including their conversation about weddings. Molly asked her if she could have a chair at the front of the church, so she could be at my level and look me in the eyes when we said our "I do's." She really was in love with me! At first, I didn't want to talk to Maggie anymore and thought it was the only way I could get over Molly, but she needed a friend, and it does warm my heart to sometimes reminisce about Molly.

Of course, I feel horrible about how I handled Molly's friends now, but from my perspective, things just seemed off. First, the only physical address I had on Molly was her friend's address. Also, I never heard her voice, and she was always reluctant to actually meet me. I had always told her the only reason we wouldn't work out would be if she were a different person from the pictures because that would mean she'd lied to me the whole time. It goes back to the first theory when she emailed me. She had to be a man, a prisoner, or a crazy woman with a wheelchair fetish. As she got to know me, she realized that I would never accept her if she were a different person. She knew that honesty was the most important thing to me and that I don't like to have people in my life I can't trust. With all these assumptions running through my mind, how could I not react the way I did?

However, I made the same mistake that we all make in society, when something happens that goes against our plans - we immediately go to the negative assumptions. It was easy for me to get down on myself again saying that all women were going to lie to me and never look past my disability. Or that this woman even had to fake her own death to get out of my life. Then the worst feeling was that I was extremely stupid for getting so wrapped up in a woman who may or may not have even been real. I am a mature, well-educated man, so how could I let myself fall for that?

I thought that I needed closure to make one of these negative thoughts a reality, but why? What would it accomplish to find out Molly was a scam? Would I have tracked her down and screamed at her? Should I meet her in a parking lot and beat her up for hurting me? No, I would never do anything like that to a person, so why not look at the positives of one of the best relationships I have ever had?

I realized the true closure I needed was to look at myself as a man and realize that I was good enough for someone to truly love me. That was Molly's gift to me. She didn't take my heart and break it. By coming into my life, she rebuilt my heart and allowed me to look past my own self-confidence issues and see the wonderful people that are still in this world. I came to this conclusion by finally accepting her death. I then looked back over our entire relationship to prove to myself that she was real.

First, I don't believe our relationship was a scam because it took way too long. I'm not sure a con artist would invest over a year in a project and never get anything out of a person. Molly never gave me an address where I could send a birthday card or any type of gift; she couldn't have been after my money. However, if it had been a scam, she definitely had plenty of opportunities to ask me for money. She could have asked for money to get home from the first accident or to help pay for cancer treatments. Maggie could have asked for help covering the funeral costs. I never received any requests for money, so if it had it been a scam, then it was a huge boost to my confidence that I made a con artist fall in love with me enough that she couldn't rip me off. Although I know in my heart Molly was real, it is pretty cool to think I might have reformed con artists.

Furthermore, Molly's story never changed. I was never able to catch her in a lie no matter how hard I tried in the beginning of our relationship when I wasn't sure if I could trust her. Unfortunately, in my rage while dealing with her death, I deleted all the emails and pictures I had from Molly, so I couldn't use them to look back over our conversations for holes that might prove she wasn't real. There was no need to do that, though. Molly meant the world to me, and I could remember everything she ever said to me. I actually paid attention to her thoughts and listened when she spoke, which is something we should all do in our relationships. Looking back on our conversations in my mind, I knew there were no holes and that she was real.

Finally, our overall connection proved that Molly was real. Although I never actually saw Molly, we shared a connection stronger than I have ever shared with a woman. We shared our innermost feelings, hopes, and dreams. We were able to come home and tell each other about our days, and we were able to work each other through our personal problems. We truly became best friends. Our relationship was a little unorthodox, but I believe we can all look at our experience to learn about our own relationships.

The only part that was missing in our relationship was the physical aspect, which I believe is part of why most relationships don't work today. Too often the physical part comes first and couples don't take the time to actually get to know each other. Too much emphasis is now placed on how "good" someone performs in the bedroom. Some men don't even know what their girlfriend's favorite flower is, but they know what alcoholic beverage puts them in the "mood." Until then, the girl is arm candy for him to show off to his buddies. Molly's favorite flower was the tulip, but she started leaning toward the purple rose because it reminded her of me. The purple rose symbolizes royalty, and she said I always made her feel like a queen. Something like that stays with a man a lot longer than a one night stand with a girl he meets in a bar.

And for that I was thankful.

Chapter 32

TESTING THE THEORY

I'VE ALWAYS HAD A THEORY that confidence is what makes a guy attractive to a woman. Not arrogance, but the confidence to overcome the fear of rejection. I believe athletes prove this theory because more often than not, the jock gets the girl. I don't believe it's because they're better men than the non-athletic person or the fact that they have great bodies or fame. I believe it's because athletes are trained to be fearless and "shake off" failures. A successful baseball player actually fails 7 out of 10 times to have a .300 batting average. A star hockey player may take 500 shots on goal in a season, but only score 50 goals. Yet, with a 10% success rate, he's probably one of the highest paid players in the league. If athletes use the same law of averages on dating as they do with sports, then they'll definitely have success dating because they aren't afraid of rejection.

I was curious to see if the same theory held true as to why Molly and I worked out so well. I was fearless in my pursuit of Molly because there were no consequences if she rejected me. I never had to actually see her, so the fears of rejection and embarrassment were gone. For my own peace of mind, I put the theory to the test after her death by joining an online dating site. It was my final test to determine not only that Molly was real, but that the love we shared was real as well. I wanted to be sure that it wasn't just me being fearless that made us work.

I actually joined two sites. I put my picture with my wheelchair on one and didn't on the other. Can you see where I was going with this experiment? On the site with my picture, I sent a few emails to women I thought I'd like to talk to. I wasn't actually looking for a new love interest, but I also knew that Molly would want me to be happy, so I had an open mind about the whole experience. On this particular site, the email recipient actually had a choice of whether or not to even read your email. They looked at your profile and made their choice then. I never even had a chance to talk to most of the people. Some were curious enough to actually read the email I sent, but I received no replies. They saw the wheelchair and didn't want to bother. I learned that people on dating sites are looking for that "fantasy" guy and that nobody's fairy tale begins with a guy with a disability. I have no ill will toward these people because of that. They just have their expectations set high with a high emphasis on physical appearance, and I can't blame them for that. We all want what we want.

On the other site, I didn't have a picture, but in my emails to people, I'd tell them to check out the hockey team website to find information on me. I was going to hide the fact that I was in a wheelchair for this part of the test, but I didn't have the heart to do it. There was still a chance that I could meet another sweet girl like Molly during this project, and it wasn't right to start it off with a lie. In the end, it didn't matter though because, again, there was no interest from the people I emailed.

The experiment proved two points. Number one was that dating sites are virtual bars, and you meet the same type of people on them as you would in a bar. For someone with a disability, our odds of getting a fair shot with a girl are just as bad on a dating site as they are in a bar. The only advantage is that you can lie about the disability on a dating site, but how are you going to handle that when you actually meet the person? Will you become belligerent when she freaks out because she didn't know you were in a chair? Will you blame her for not treating you fairly when you lied to her from the beginning? Personally, I wouldn't blame a girl for leaving if I did that to her. My best advice is to be honest from the beginning about everything.

The second point proven from my experiment was that Molly truly loved me for the person I had become. I took the same approach with the dating sites that I had when she and I first starting talking to each other but had completely different results. The dating site experiment was a hit to my confidence because I thought I had finally figured out how to talk to women. It was also extremely gratifying to finally accept that someone truly loved me.

I hoped I could find that again.

Chapter 33

❧

MOLLY'S PURPOSE

WHILE I'M SAD ABOUT MOLLY'S death, I'm not angry; in fact, I'm grateful. Molly was sent to me in a time of need; by the time she left this world, she had rekindled my faith in mankind. In a time where we focus on the negative, Molly showed me that there are still good people in this world. On Molly's social networking site, she had a quote that she said was meant for me. It said, "If I could sit on the porch across from God, I would thank Him for lending me you." Ironically, it was she that was lent to me.

When we first started talking to each other, one of her questions was about my life expectancy. Of course, I couldn't answer that. All I knew was that the doctors told my parents I wouldn't live past the age of two. Lucky for me, they got a second opinion, and I am (obviously) still here today. I did tell Molly that nobody knew how long they were going to be on this Earth. God didn't create us with expiration dates. All we can do is live life to the fullest while we can. It was strange to me how I had to "practice what I was preaching" after her untimely death.

There was a time when I was a little angry with God for taking Molly away after I was certain He brought her into my life. People have asked me if I was angry with God for putting me here with a disability, but I never have been. I believe while He didn't make me physically strong enough to do much of anything, He made me emotionally strong enough to handle everything. If by having a disability, I can help others appreciate what they have, then I think I'm doing my job while I'm here. With everything I go through in a day, if I can maintain my positive outlook on life, then the average Joe is able to see that his "problems" are really quite small.

Could I inspire others if I were "normal?" Perhaps if I ended up being a professional athlete or something, but how could the drive and desire I have now be guaranteed if life was easy? Personally, I believe God made me the way He wanted me, and I have no problem being different. Molly and I actually began to realize that being "abnormal" was a compliment. She was definitely not a normal woman, but as I told her, "Anyone can be normal, I would much rather have someone who is extraordinary."

So why did Molly have to leave? I believe that she had done her job. When I asked for her to come into my life, I didn't ask for a lifetime of happiness with her, I asked for a woman to be honest with me and that I would take care of the rest. I don't believe God is that literal with our prayers, but maybe Molly wasn't "the one" for me. While I have a really hard time with that thought because I could definitely see us growing old together, I also refuse to believe that I can never find another love.

In a time when I was about ready to give up on certain things in life and just accept that I wouldn't be able to live all my dreams, Molly showed up and reminded me that I could have everything that I ever wanted. I just had to be patient and continue my relentless pursuit of those goals. Molly showed me that I was right in the pursuit of my idea of "perfection" when it came to choosing a significant other. She proved that I was good enough for a great person to fall in love with, and I am now confident that it can happen again.

We should all have such confidence. In other aspects of our life we don't accept mediocrity, or at least we shouldn't. We go to school to pursue college and then pursue a career. We don't work for all those years in the classroom to be stuck in a job we hate for 30 years; we do it because we dream of a better life. Why should we be any different in our pursuit of love? I wouldn't want to be stuck in a miserable marriage for 30 years because I settled.

Chapter 34

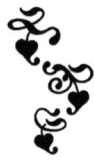

❧

REAL BEAUTY

I BELIEVE WE CAN ALL FIND that "perfect" person. We all deserve to have the "most beautiful woman in the world." I'm sure someone is reading this and saying, "But Jonathan, what about me? I'm not a super model." Yes, the girls on the covers of magazines are physically attractive, but that's all they are… an attraction. True beauty lies within a person. Yes, physical attraction gets you to talk to a person, but after you say "Hi," the true beauty comes out. They either become more beautiful every time you talk, or the attraction fades away pretty quickly.

Attraction is different for every person. We all like different things. Think of attraction like a restaurant. The signs, the building, and the atmosphere get you to the table, but it's the actual food that makes you stay or even come back to eat again. The women on the covers of magazines are just that, a sign to attract you. Market researchers know exactly what they're doing when they put certain celebrities on magazines. They have data telling them what color dress is most appealing to the public and even what angle of head turn is most attractive for that specific person. Perhaps their data is not that drastic, but the celebrities are exceptionally attractive because the advertisers want them to be.

The only difference between you and them is that their whole life is about making themselves attractive to the public. If you didn't have a 40 hour/week job, could work out with a personal trainer daily, have cosmetologists handle your makeup and hair and dieticians telling you what to eat, I'm sure you could be just as "attractive" as the cover girls. However, if you had all that, would you be truly beautiful? You may have guys fawning over you for a notch in their bed posts, but it wouldn't help you find the true love we all desire.

What makes you beautiful is already there. It's in all of us. The trick is that you have to have the confidence in yourself to let it out. Is it shallow of me to say that I won't settle for anyone less than the most beautiful girl in the world? No, I don't think so because when I do find that special lady, she will be the most beautiful girl in the world to me. Would she be on the cover of a magazine? I don't know, but in my eyes she could be.

Looking back at Molly, she did become that woman for me. Every time we talked, she became more beautiful to me, and I became more handsome to her. By talking online daily and truly getting to know each other, we provided the substance in our relationship that kept us coming back to each other. Communication was the food that fed our relationship. When we are old and our looks fade, all we will have to fall back on is the ability to talk to the person we're spending our life with, so it's probably a good idea to have common interests and beliefs.

Our relationship worked because we communicated. We didn't worry about being politically correct or offending each other. Yes, she had questions specifically about my disability, which were easy to answer, but we all have concerns that we may be hiding because of fear of offending the other person. For example, I believe it's important to find out about religious beliefs of a person. You don't have to be a minister or go to church every Sunday because I don't make it every week myself, but I do want to be with someone who believes in the same God I do.

Also, family questions are important. Some people avoid these, but it's good to know if their parents are divorced, how their parents raised them, etc. Our parents help us become the adults we are, so asking about family is a good way to get a background on someone. I was always told to look at a woman's mother because that is who she will become. I don't believe they'll become mirror images of their mothers, but I do believe a mother will instill the same values on her daughter. Overall, by asking questions we were able to learn about each other and build a stronger relationship.

We also never "went to bed angry," although it did take us a few days at times to get our thoughts together to work out our dis-agreements. When we did have our problems, we talked through them. By talking through them, I don't mean we argued until we had a winner. We listened to both sides, and we both apologized. Our apologies were sincere, and we never had the same problems again. Rather than allow a disagreement to wound our relation-ship and keep picking at the "scab," we took the time to make sure we healed the wound.

While communication is the key to a successful relationship, good communication goes back to being fearless in the relationship. The bottom line is that a person will either want a relationship with you, or they won't. In the end it is, and always will be, their choice. The best thing you can do is show them your true self by not being afraid to give honest answers. Molly and I were able to do this without hesitation because we knew life wouldn't be over if our online relationship didn't work out. We would be disap-pointed, but life would go on as it always does. Too often, people adapt their values or beliefs because they're afraid to lose a person. This simply cannot be done if you want to have a successful rela-tionship with someone. If you don't like sushi, say you don't like sushi, don't fake it just to make her think you have something in common. If something that small causes a relationship to end, then you were better off single.

I firmly believe honesty truly is the best policy.

Chapter 35

❧

FINDING YOURSELF

*H*AVE YOU EVER SEEN A couple in public and said, "Wow how did that guy get a girl like that?" I imagine we've all said that at one time or another. I know I have. We often follow that question with, "I'll never get a girl like her." In order to find love, you first have to love yourself. If you don't think that you are worth that "perfect" person, then you're right. True beauty lies within you. It is your job to bring it to the surface so that "perfect" person can see it. If you don't have the confidence to be yourself, then that person will not give you the attention you desire. Maybe they still won't be interested after you approach them and show them the real you, but you may discover that you aren't interested in them, either.

The right people fit together. It will just happen. You can't build anything on lies; you have to be yourself. So why did that guy end up with that girl? Because she met him before she met you. He doesn't have anything more to offer her than you already have. You have to believe in yourself and never settle for less than the best for you.

I never understood the old adage, "it is better to have loved and lost than to never have loved at all," before I met Molly. After my experience with her, the adage holds true. Yes, losing her caused great heartache, but she changed my whole outlook on life. I am definitely a better person overall because of Molly. I will never forget my online angel and will be eternally grateful for all the gifts she gave me in our short time together.

I hope that one day another angel will come into my life.

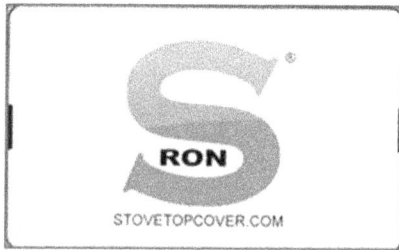

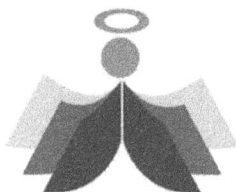

MilversteadPublishing

Our books are bound by commitment.

To learn more about our commitment to bringing
great books to market while helping good causes,
please visit us on the web at
http://www.milversteadpublishing.com

www.ingramcontent.com/pod-product-compliance
Lightning Source LLC
Chambersburg PA
CBHW021341290326
41933CB00037B/318